MODERNIZING MEDICARE

modernizing medicare

HARNESSING
THE POWER OF
CONSUMER CHOICE
AND MARKET
COMPETITION

EDITED BY
ROBERT EMMET MOFFIT
MARIE FISHPAW

JOHNS HOPKINS UNIVERSITY PRESS | *Baltimore*

© 2023 The Heritage Foundation
All rights reserved. Published 2023
Printed in the United States of America on acid-free paper
2 4 6 8 9 7 5 3 1

Johns Hopkins University Press
2715 North Charles Street
Baltimore, Maryland 21218
www.press.jhu.edu

Cataloging-in-Publication Data is available from the Library of Congress.

A catalog record for this book is available from the British Library.

ISBN: 978-1-4214-4602-8 (hardcover)
ISBN: 978-1-4214-4603-5 (ebook)

Special discounts are available for bulk purchases of this book. For more information, please contact Special Sales at specialsales@jh.edu.

CONTENTS

CONTRIBUTORS

EDITORS

Robert Emmet Moffit, PhD
Senior Fellow in Domestic
	Policy Studies
The Heritage Foundation
Washington, DC

Marie Fishpaw
Independent Domestic Policy
	Consultant
Washington, DC

AUTHORS

Joseph R. Antos, PhD
Senior Fellow and Wilson H. Taylor
	Scholar in Health Care and
	Retirement Policy
American Enterprise Institute
Washington, DC

Doug Badger
Senior Fellow at the Galen Institute
	and Senior Fellow at the Heritage
	Foundation
Ponte Vedra, Florida

Charles P. Blahous, PhD
J. Fish and Lillian F. Smith Chair
	and Senior Research Strategist
Mercatus Center

George Mason University
Fairfax, Virginia

Walton J. Francis
Independent Economist and
	Consultant
Fairfax, Virginia

John C. Goodman, PhD
President
Goodman Institute for Public Policy
	Research
Dallas, Texas

Edmund F. Haislmaier
Preston A. Wells, Jr., Senior Research
	Fellow in Domestic Policy Studies
The Heritage Foundation
Washington, DC

Douglas Holtz-Eakin, PhD
President
American Action Forum
Washington, DC

Brian J. Miller, MD, MBA, MPH
Assistant Professor of Medicine and
	Business
Johns Hopkins University
Baltimore, Maryland

Mark V. Pauly, PhD
Professor Emeritus in the Department
  of Health Care Management
The Wharton School
University of Pennsylvania
Philadelphia, Pennsylvania

Christopher Pope, PhD
Senior Fellow
Manhattan Institute
New York, New York

Gail R. Wilensky, PhD
Senior Fellow
Project Hope
Bethesda, Maryland

MODERNIZING MEDICARE

Introduction

Reviving the Medicare Reform Consensus

In 1996, the editors of the *New York Times* hailed a "new consensus" on the future of Medicare:

> When it was created in the 1960s, Medicare gave the elderly the same fee-for-service coverage that everyone else used. But now Medicare stands nearly alone in providing the most expensive health care choice, at huge taxpayer expense. One result has been a growing consensus among ideologically diverse people that the structure of Medicare must change. The list of reformers includes Nancy Johnson, the House Republican from Connecticut; Ron Wyden, a Senate Democrat from Oregon; the Brookings Institution, a liberal leaning think tank; and the Heritage Foundation, a conservative think tank. The latest addition to the list is the American Medical Association, the physicians' group that tried to scuttle Medicare at its inception.[1]

The *Times'* editors neatly summarized the fundamental point of this remarkable bipartisan consensus:

> Their proposal mirrors the market-based system that gives millions of federal employees a wide range of choice of health plans. It allows the

1

elderly to stick with the traditional fee-for-service government-run program, a deft political stroke that could take the fear out of reform for many elderly. Retirees could choose instead a private managed care plan that offers additional benefits, like coverage for drugs or lower fees. They would pay more for expensive plans and receive rebates for choosing inexpensive plans.

These defined contribution advocates soon made some progress. The Balanced Budget Act of 1997 created the National Bipartisan Commission on the Future of Medicare, chaired by Sen. John Breaux (D-LA) and Rep. William Thomas (R-CA and chairman of the House Committee on Ways and Means).[2] In 1999, the majority of that commission proposed transforming Medicare into a "premium support" system of financing[3] while also restructuring it based on the Federal Employees Health Benefits Program. While the Breaux-Thomas recommendation failed to command the support of either the Clinton administration or Congress, the Bush administration succeeded in making a big step in its direction by enacting the Medicare Modernization Act of 2003 and creating Medicare Advantage and Medicare Part D, the prescription drug program. Both programs were systems of competing private plans, and both, though differently structured, were financed on a defined contribution basis.

In 2012, Rep. Paul Ryan (R-WI) and Sen. Ron Wyden (D-OR) revived the premium support proposal, and the bipartisan idea again attracted staunch support within Washington's diverse policy community.[4] The Wyden-Ryan proposal, however, faced inveterate opposition from the Obama administration and its congressional allies.

The Impending Financial Crisis

Medicare is facing an immediate fiscal challenge. The Medicare Board of Trustees reports that the Medicare Hospital Insurance (HI) Trust Fund, the account for Part A hospital and related medical services, will be insolvent in 2028.[5]

Insolvency in this Medicare context, incidentally, does not mean "bankruptcy" in the sense of a total financial collapse, the sort of catastrophe that destroys a private sector firm. Rather, it means that the Medicare hospital insurance program will not be able to pay for all the promised Medicare Part A benefits. The timing of trust fund insolvency is, of course, dependent upon economic conditions and payroll tax revenues. The anticipated Medicare hospital payment reduction, assuming trust fund exhaustion in 2028, would initially amount to 10 percent,[6] and, absent remedial action, the annual payment cuts would continue and progressively deepen thereafter. Such reductions in payment for medical services, the Medicare trustees warn, would directly hurt the beneficiaries dependent on those services: "Beneficiary access to health care services could be rapidly curtailed."[7]

The HI trust fund, declare the trustees, meets neither their short-term nor long-term standards of financial adequacy, meaning that its assets should equal 100 percent of its annual expenditures. Except for just two years (2016 and 2017), Part A spending exceeded income since 2008. At the beginning of 2022, Part A assets amounted to just 40 percent of the hospital expenditures projected for the year.[8]

Part A insolvency has never occurred in the history of the Medicare program. The congressional options to prevent it are, however, both limited and painful: an increase in the federal payroll tax, a new charge on Medicare beneficiaries, a transfer of general revenues into the HI trust fund, likely meaning higher income or business taxes. Otherwise, they may resort to some new set of Medicare price controls or payment reductions for Medicare Part A providers, already subject to hundreds of billions of dollars in payment reductions for the foreseeable future under the Affordable Care Act of 2010.

Outdated Model

Enacted in 1965, Medicare was designed as a defined benefit, fee-for-service program for hospital (Part A) and physicians (Part B) services. Since its inception, original Medicare's basic structure remained largely the same, though Congress enacted significant changes in provider payment.

Medicare's benefit delivery options, however, *did* change, and in a major way. Building on limited experimentation with health maintenance organizations (HMOs) in the early 1970s, Congress enacted the Tax Equity and Fiscal Responsibility Act of 1982, and codified private HMOs as an alternative (Medicare Part C) to traditional Medicare.[9] Because the HMOs failed to deliver anticipated savings, however, Congress created "Medicare+Choice" as part of the Balanced Budget Act of 1997. That law added preferred provider organizations as an option and allowed plans to offer benefits beyond Part A and B categories, permitting the plans to charge additional premiums for the additional benefits. Nonetheless, excessive regulation and inadequate health plan payment led to a drop in plan participation and enrollment. Congress reversed course with the enactment of the Medicare Modernization Act of 2003 and renamed the alternative private-plan program "Medicare Advantage." The law changed the plan payment formula and established a new risk adjustment system, expanded plan options and permitted more varied benefit offerings, and created a new "rebate" system to secure savings to beneficiaries (and the government) if they purchased efficient plans. The 2003 law thus established the Medicare Advantage program as we know it today.

Though Medicare's benefit delivery through private plans changed over the years, Medicare's fee-for-service system is, and has been, facing deepening financial troubles. Today, the impending Part A financial crisis should encourage a rethinking of traditional social insurance, the conceptual basis of both Medicare and Social Security. The traditional concept of social insurance is based on the principal that the beneficiaries should pay for the benefits they get. The payroll tax imposed during the working life of beneficiaries is the mechanism for that payment. In the case of Medicare Part A, a classic social insurance model, Congress established a "pay-as-you-go" system, meaning that today's nonworking retirees are supported by today's workers, just as yesterday's retirees were supported by yesterday's workers.

The affordability of such a model is heavily dependent upon the nation's demographics; ideally, a relatively large number of workers supporting a smaller number of beneficiaries. In the United States, and in many other countries, a major demographic shift, particularly the rapid aging and extended longevity of the population, has altered the demographic balance. In the case of Medicare, for example, beneficiary enrollment has doubled over the past 35 years, and the Medicare trustees project it will grow by 50 percent over the next 35 years. At the same time, however, the number of workers supporting the number of beneficiaries is shrinking. In 2008, there were four workers to each Medicare beneficiary, but by 2019 there were just three workers to each beneficiary. By 2030, when the baby boom generation is fully retired, there will be only 2.5 workers supporting each Medicare beneficiary.[10]

Spending Growth

Threats to the solvency of the Part A trust fund are a marker of a much larger problem: the rapid and consuming growth in Medicare spending. While Medicare Part A is racing toward insolvency, Medicare Parts B and D, the supplementary medical insurance (SMI) program, also faces fiscal challenges. In 2020, Part B benefit costs alone grew at a rate of 13.2 percent, reflecting the massive increase in COVID-19 spending.[11] For the next ten years, the cost for SMI (Parts B and D combined) is projected to grow at an average annual rate of 8 percent, much faster than the growth of wages or the general economy and reflective of the retirement of the big baby boom generation.[12] As a share of the gross domestic product (GDP), Part B spending alone amounted to 1.88 percent of GDP in 2020, but it is projected to reach 3.29 percent by 2040.[13]

While beneficiary SMI premiums fund about a quarter of benefits and services, automatic drawdowns of general revenues (funded by business and income taxes) account for roughly three-fourths of spending. For beneficiaries, SMI premiums and cost sharing are projected to consume 28 percent of beneficiaries' average Social Security benefit in 2022.[14] For taxpayers, SMI premiums consumed 17 percent of all business and income taxes in 2019, but they are projected to consume 21.5 percent by 2030 and 26.6 percent by 2040.[15]

Under current law, if general revenues to fund Medicare exceed 45 percent of total Medicare spending twice within seven years, the trustees must issue a formal Medicare funding warning.[16] The president and Congress are legally obliged to take remedial action. While the trustees have issued multiple warnings, thus far neither presidents nor lawmakers have taken remedial action.

Future Debt

It is very likely that the next major debate on the future of Medicare will take place within the context of multi-trillion-dollar annual deficits, dangerous levels of debt, and perhaps even the threat of a fiscal crisis.[17] Congress's multi-trillion-dollar pandemic spending has already added to the nation's record debt: over $31 trillion (about $95,000 per person in the United States). Long-term (over the next 75 years), Medicare is generating huge unfunded obligations, which are the total cost of promised Medicare benefits that are not financed either by dedicated revenues or beneficiary premiums. The trustees note that the HI portion of these obligations ($5.1 trillion) are likely to be addressed by future legislation or expenditure cuts, but the SMI portion ($47.5 trillion) "will require general fund transfers of this amount, and these transfers represent a formal budget requirement."[18] In short, Medicare's unfunded obligations will amount to $52.6 trillion (about $160,000 per person in the United States), another future taxpayer burden dwarfing America's rapidly rising national debt.[19]

Harnessing the Power of Choice and Competition

While many of Washington's progressive politicians are committed to abolishing private and employer-based health insurance altogether,[20] others wish to overhaul health care financing and delivery based on government central planning and price regulation, heavier insurance regulation, and larger taxpayer subsidies.[21]

These progressive proposals for stronger federal government control are countered by a growing bipartisan commitment to choice and competition in health reform. For example, state and federal policymakers, on a bipartisan basis, are demonstrating an increasing commitment to transparency in price and provider performance, taking advantage of waivers from federal mandates to lower insurance costs, while providing greater opportunities for convenient and personalized delivery of care through direct primary care programs and a wider availability of telehealth.[22] In recent years, the United States has also experienced a growing expansion of consumer decision-making, evident in the rapid growth of health savings accounts, health reimbursement accounts, and flexible spending accounts.

Alternative Vision

When it comes to Medicare's future, there are rational alternatives to resolving the program's many problems by merely raising taxes, tightening price controls, or cutting provider payments for Medicare benefits and services. While the authors of this volume do not agree on all the technical details of reform, they strongly agree that Washington policymakers can and should harness the enormous power of consumer choice and genuine market competition.

The best mechanism for harnessing that power is the defined contribution system of financing. In its most basic form, the government makes an annual per capita contribution to a health plan of a beneficiary's choice. The dollar amount of that government contribution is set by a benchmark, which is itself the product of a market-based bid (a competitive bid) among competing health plans. If a beneficiary chooses a health plan that is more expensive than the government contribution, the beneficiary pays the difference in a higher premium for enrolling in that plan. If the beneficiary chooses a health plan whose premium costs are below the government's benchmark contribution, the beneficiary can keep the difference in the form of personal savings.

To a degree, Medicare already embodies this financing approach. Medicare Advantage, the system of competing private health plans, is a defined contribution program largely (though not entirely) based on market-driven competitive bidding. Medicare Advantage has enjoyed stunning growth in recent years, and the Medicare trustees estimate that the program will enroll over 30 million beneficiaries, accounting for 46.2 percent of total Medicare enrollment, in 2022.[23] Likewise, Medicare Part D, the Medicare prescription drug program, is a defined contribution system in which drugs are delivered through competing private plans. That approach is remarkably similar to the Federal Employees Health Benefits Program (FEHBP) in its financing.

The popular and successful Federal Employees Health Benefits Program, which has been operating for over six decades, also offers a sound model for the administration and the light and flexible regulation of a large defined contribution system. Serving over 8 million federal employees, retirees, and their families, the program contracts with hundreds of plans in states, and there are normally about 20 plans serving beneficiaries in all counties throughout the United States.

During the mid-1990s, as noted, the FEHBP emerged as a preferred model for reforming Medicare. In 1999, the FEHBP became the model for the majority recommendation of the National Bipartisan Commission on the Future of Medicare (the Breaux-Thomas commission).[24]

Improving the Medicare Advantage Program

Traditional Medicare and Medicare Advantage, as well as their constituent features of finance and delivery, present a rich field for research and analysis as well as opportunities for policy innovation.[25] While the contributing authors of this book share a common conviction in the general superiority of market forces in the financing and delivery of health benefits and services, they do not all agree on specific policy measures. This is especially true of certain technical issues, fraught with the potential for unintended consequences, such as how best to refine or restructure Medicare's risk adjustment system or how to devise the best formula for government contributions to health plans on behalf of beneficiaries. Such differences invite further empirical analyses and should encourage rigorous testing and demonstration projects.

Improving Medicare Advantage and, beyond that, harnessing choice and competition in a comprehensive Medicare reform, would require significant policy changes. The authors address these changes in their essays.

Tackling the Tough Task of Reform

In chapter 2, Professor Mark V. Pauly, PhD, of the University of Pennsylvania addresses the daunting challenge of reforming the almost 60-year-old Medicare fee-for-service (FFS) program. Assessing the reform prospects from a "public choice" perspective—the application of economic analysis to political decisions—Pauly concludes that for the foreseeable future the program will remain hard to reform if voters, rightly or wrongly, perceive proposed improvements as incompatible with their self-interest. In this volume, as Pauly notes, the authors value reform to improve the program for beneficiaries, viewing the decline in spending growth as a beneficial, though crucial, byproduct of these improvements. Absent reform, however, the "chickens will come home to roost" in the form of higher taxes, larger deficits, and bigger debt. If, and when, voters are negatively impacted by these consequences, their calculations may change, and they may perhaps realize that reform based on the principles of choice and competition is the "better path" for Medicare's future and their own.

Reforming amid Financial Crisis

Against the backdrop of the pending trust fund insolvency, former Medicare trustee Charles P. Blahous, PhD, emphasizes in chapter 3 that the bigger problem is that Americans are being made "poorer" by the federal government's failure to contain health care costs, especially the rising costs of Medicare. In fact, the supplementary medical insurance program is a significantly bigger problem for taxpayers than the financial shortfalls facing the hospital insurance trust fund. This situation, according to Blahous, requires policymakers to think big: "The irony is that Medicare as we know it cannot be preserved unless it is significantly changed."

Among the "daunting" financial numbers, Blahous highlights a "pocket" of good news: the performance of the Medicare Advantage program. Medicare Advantage has not only experienced phenomenal growth, far surpassing the expectations of the Medicare trustees, but it has demonstrated that it can reduce the costs of delivering the standard Part A and Part B benefits. While "past performance is no guarantee of future results," Medicare Advantage's performance is grounds for optimism, an approach that can secure excellent value for increasingly precious health care dollars.

A Record of Success

In chapter 4, Christopher Pope, PhD, senior fellow at the Manhattan Institute, describes the remarkable success of Medicare Advantage. That success is evident in its rapid expansion, broad range of choice and competition, and its competitive pricing of benefits and services. The program's rapid enrollment growth has been matched by an increase in choice of plans and the continuous provision of benefits and services at competitive premiums.

Given its sheer size, traditional Medicare has an enormous influence on health care financing, pricing, and care delivery in the commercial insurance markets and on Medicare Advantage itself, where provider prices often shadow its complex system of administrative payment and price controls. Although traditional Medicare can secure hospital services at lower prices than commercial insurance, Pope observes, the more flexible Medicare Advantage plans are nonetheless able to negotiate "a better deal" than traditional Medicare.

According to government actuaries, beneficiaries enrolled in Medicare Advantage plans saved $1.5 billion in their premium costs between 2017 and 2020.[26] Medicare Advantage plans have been able to deliver the standard Medicare Part A and B benefits at less cost than Medicare FFS, says Pope, and he shows how Medicare Advantage stacks up against Medicare FFS in specific benefit and services cost comparisons. He reveals how Medicare Advantage's more flexible payment arrangements stimulate innovation in care delivery, noting that Medicare Advantage plans focus heavily on preventative care and thus secure a wide variety of medical outcomes that are superior to those of beneficiaries enrolled in traditional Medicare.

Personalized Care

While Pope emphasizes Medicare Advantage's impressive record of success, in chapter 5, John C. Goodman, PhD, the "father of health savings accounts," outlines a series of recommendations to enable the program to perform even better. Noting that Medicare Advantage has been "immensely successful," Goodman says that far too many bureaucratic and regulatory barriers remain and that Washington policymakers should unleash the power of patients—as consumers of medical goods and services—to achieve higher-quality care and save money in the process.

To begin, Goodman calls for changes to get sick patients access to better care and additional choices, starting by eliminating restrictions on the ability of senior citizens to make deposits in tax-free health savings accounts or to have health reimbursement accounts outside of the employer-based health insurance system. For chronically ill patients, Goodman argues for the creation of a stand-alone health savings accounts, disconnected from third party insurance. A good model for this arrangement, he notes, is the successful Medicaid "cash and counseling" program, whereby patients and their caregivers were able to manage their own budgets with a high degree of flexibility to secure the care they need, when they need it, and from the medical professional best able to provide it.

Goodman makes several other recommendations, such as allowing Medicare patients and their doctors to take full advantage of telehealth, integrating direct primary care into the Medicare program, allowing Medicare Advantage plans to provide financial incentives to patients who adopt healthy behavior, and improving Medicare Advantage's risk adjustment to facilitate the ability of patients to switch health plans to secure the best quality of care for their medical condition.

Accelerating Enrollment

While Goodman charts a path for patient power as the key to improving the program's performance, in chapter 6, Johns Hopkins University hospitalist Brian J. Miller, MD, and former Medicare administrator Gail R. Wilensky, PhD, argue that Congress should take the next rational step: make Medicare Advantage enrollment the default enrollment for new Medicare beneficiaries.

When it comes to beneficiary enrollment, there is no "level playing field" between traditional Medicare and Medicare Advantage plans. Currently, Medicare beneficiaries are automatically enrolled in the Medicare FFS and are subject to a financial penalty for late enrollment. Miller and Wilensky call for a reversal of this process, without the penalty. While beneficiaries would, of course, be free to withdraw from the Medicare Advantage plan and enroll instead in traditional Medicare, automatic enrollment in private retirement programs routinely demonstrates a high rate of continued participation and would further accelerate the expansion of private plan enrollment among Medicare beneficiaries.

For Miller and Wilensky, these changes would represent an organic evolution, as Medicare Advantage to date has offered a "natural experiment" in health plan competition and is delivering on its promise of providing value for health care dollars. The authors conclude that Medicare Advantage default enrollment also would establish the groundwork for a comprehensive reform of the Medicare program based on defined contribution (premium support) financing. If Congress were to switch to auto-enrollment of new beneficiaries into Medicare Advantage rather than traditional Medicare, they argue, lawmakers would not only harness market-based incentives for controlling the overall growth of Medicare spending, but they would also stimulate innovation in benefit design and value-based care delivery. This change would secure major advantages for beneficiaries and taxpayers alike.

In short, the Medicare Advantage default enrollment proposal, advanced by Wilensky and Miller, would serve as a *transitional* mechanism in the evolution of Medicare toward a fully defined contribution (premium support) program. When there is direct competition among all health plans, including an updated Medicare fee-for-service plan, the maintenance of a level playing field (i.e., the absence of any statutory or regulatory advantage for any competing plan) would be an essential condition of that competition.

Transitioning to Comprehensive Premium Support

The goal of true comprehensive Medicare reform should be to give every beneficiary the personal choice of their health plan and create a competitive system of plans and providers that will enable beneficiaries to secure the best value for their Medicare dollars. The best means to accomplish this goal is to build on the existing infrastructure of Medicare Advantage and require traditional Medicare to compete, while improving Medicare Advantage's key features, including the plan payment and risk adjustment systems.

Building on Medicare Advantage's Infrastructure

In chapter 7, I outline the key tasks that must be undertaken to transform Medicare into a comprehensive and fully competitive premium support system based on the existing infrastructure of the Medicare

Advantage program: a well-established working model of a defined contribution (premium support) system.

Citing Medicare Advantage's success—particularly its rapid enrollment growth and its delivery of benefits and services at competitive prices—I maintain Medicare Advantage is the ideal platform for comprehensive change and emphasize that effecting such a major transition would require significant modifications in Medicare Advantage's structure and operations.

To start, the entire program must be competitive on a level playing field with a common set of rules. I argue that Medicare FFS itself must be compelled to compete, and to secure that robust competition, Medicare FFS must be updated: it should deliver benefits through a modern, integrated plan design rather than as a disjointed set of benefit categories based on a 1960s insurance model. Such a reform would allow the traditional program to compete directly with private health plans.

Functionally, the government plan payment systems, including risk adjustment payment, must also be overhauled. The federal government's *per capita* contribution to health plans should be simplified and based on market-based competitive bidding. The Medicare Advantage risk adjustment system, which has been improved in recent years, must be improved even more; it must target health risk more accurately and effectively and prevent the billions of dollars' worth of health plan gaming at the expense of the taxpayers.

I also recommend that Medicare's complex and cumbersome regulatory system should be thoroughly renovated and refocused on consumer protection. Executive branch officials should be prevented from interfering with a normal market interaction between competing private health plans and providers over benefit options, medical practice guidelines, or pricing for medical services. Such regulatory reform, accompanied by a reduction in the power of the Medicare bureaucracy, would allow for the full flowering of the innovation in benefit design, provider payment arrangements, and more personalized health care delivery.

In chapter 8, Joseph R. Antos, PhD, former assistant director of the nonpartisan Congressional Budget Office (CBO) and currently a senior fellow at the American Enterprise Institute, takes a closer look at what is needed to modernize and upgrade the traditional Medicare FFS program.

Antos recognizes that the continued existence of traditional Medicare would not only enhance beneficiary choice, allowing those who are comfortable with the fee-for service system to remain with it, but such robust private plan competition with the traditional Medicare would improve its performance and could also generate positive fiscal consequences.[27]

Antos suggests integrating Medicare Part A and B into a single comprehensive health benefits program, reforming and streamlining the complicated cost-sharing arrangements of the traditional program, and adding a hard cap on beneficiaries' out of pocket expenses, thus securing the fundamental purpose of health insurance: protection of beneficiaries from the financial devastation of catastrophic illness. Antos says that such a change should be accompanied by new managerial flexibility to enable the FFS program to compete effectively with private plans in a dynamic health insurance market. This would not only secure a level playing field between Medicare FFS and private health plans—the *sine qua non* of free and fair market competition—but it would also reduce beneficiaries' dependence on costly supplemental insurance, increase the efficiency of the geographical markets, relieve Medicare beneficiaries of the financial burdens of paying additional premiums, and reduce the excessive Medicare spending borne by the taxpayers.

Fixing Risk Adjustment

No health insurance market, no matter how robust initially, is immune from the threat of adverse selection. Adverse selection takes place when sicker enrollees congregate disproportionately in a health plan, driving up that plan's claims and premium costs, and progressively weakening its ability to compete in the market. The dynamics of this process, left unaddressed, result in the so-called "death spiral": rapidly rising premium costs, an increasingly concentrated market, reduced choice for enrollees, and eventually the collapse of market competition.

As part of its plan payment process, the current Medicare Advantage (MA) program has in place a risk adjustment system to prevent this market instability. As analysts with the Bipartisan Policy Center, a prominent Washington think tank, have observed, "The MA risk adjustment is the most sophisticated method in use, but it is not perfect."[28] While the federal government's base payment to Medicare Advantage plans is tied to the cost of providing Medicare's traditional benefits, the payment is also adjusted on the risk scores of actual plan enrollees, their demographic data and their medical diagnoses. In short, it is a *prospective* risk adjustment, but it fails to account adequately for the costs of sick individuals.

In chapter 9, Heritage Foundation Research Fellow Edmund F. Haislmaier proposes ways to improve the risk adjustment payments. His idea retains a *prospective* approach for adjusting plan payments to reflect nonhealth factors (geography) and enrollee demographics (age, sex). And he proposes to refine this model with the creation of a "risk transfer pool" to enable participating insurers to adjust among themselves for any selection effects. In short, the pool would operate mainly on a *retrospective* basis, and would adjust for any maldistribution of risks in the aggregate, as opposed to trying to project the costs of individual enrollees. As Haislmaier observes, such a risk-adjusted payment system would be based on hard data, not guesswork, and it would secure the affordability of premiums for enrollees and the stability of the market for competing health plans.

Improving Medicare Drug Plans

Along with Medicare Advantage, the Medicare Modernization Act of 2003 created Medicare Part D, a system of competing health plans that deliver a standard drug benefit. In chapter 10, Mr. Doug Badger, a former health policy adviser to President George W. Bush during the creation of the programs, describes Part D as the "prototype of premium support."

In Medicare Part D, the federal government's role is largely confined to making a direct contribution equal to roughly three quarters of the plan's premium costs, but the terms and conditions of drug pricing and delivery are set solely through private market negotiations between drug manufacturers and health plans. (This contrasts with Medicare Part A and B, in which the government directly sets and controls the prices for medical benefits and services.) Private market negotiations have delivered not only significant savings for taxpayers but also major savings for Medicare beneficiaries. Over the period of 2017 to 2020, for example, Medicare beneficiaries have saved an estimated $3.4 billion in premium costs.[29] Moreover, as Badger points out, the expanded provision of prescription drug therapies at competitive prices has also reduced health spending on other medical benefits and services. Assorted studies have also shown that expanded drug access has resulted in better medical outcomes for Medicare beneficiaries.

While the Medicare drug program has been successful, Badger calls attention to certain structural flaws that generate perverse incentives for drug manufacturers, health plans, and beneficiaries. He offers several recommendations to correct them, notably putting health plans and manufacturers more at risk for higher drug spending and establishing a hard cap on Medicare beneficiaries' annual out-of-pocket drug spending.

Advantages for Beneficiaries and Taxpayers

In chapter 11, Walton J. Francis, an economist specializing in health insurance and formerly a consultant on Medicare Advantage regulations for the Centers for Medicare and Medicaid Services, traces the history of Medicare premium support (the most prominent defined contribution model) through the seminal experience of the Federal Employees Health Benefit Program, created in 1960, and the Medicare Advantage program, created in 2003.

Francis emphasizes that premium support has had a strong bipartisan pedigree, championed by both liberal and conservative academics and policy analysts. While conservatives in Congress, such as former House Speaker Paul Ryan (R-WI) and former House Ways and Means Chairman Bill Thomas (R-CA), have sponsored major Medicare premium support proposals, the term "premium support" was coined by Dr. Henry Aaron of the Brookings Institution and Dr. Robert Reischauer of the Urban Institute, and this approach to comprehensive reform was endorsed by the late Alice Rivlin, former CBO director, as well as analysts with the Progressive Policy Institute.

In his essay, Francis describes how existing Medicare Advantage and FEHBP premium support works, assesses the strengths and weaknesses of the programs' current approaches, and suggests ways to improve upon the model to secure a brighter future for Medicare beneficiaries and their programs.

Savings for Beneficiaries and Taxpayers

In chapter 12, former CBO director Douglas Holtz-Eakin, PhD, estimates the potential of personal savings for Medicare beneficiaries, as well as program savings for taxpayers, in a transition to a Medicare premium support system. In his essay, Holtz-Eakin discusses the key design features that would contribute to such fiscal success, as well as evidence from the experience of Medicare Advantage and the Federal Employees Health Benefits Program, both defined contribution models of health care financing. Based on his analysis of previous CBO estimates and extrapolating from CBO baseline data, Holtz-Eakin concludes that the 10-year savings for beneficiaries and taxpayers alike would be substantial.

Looking Ahead

Previous reform efforts were stimulated by a variety of concerns: Medicare's financial challenges, the need for greater efficiency in the delivery of care, the reduction of unnecessary bureaucracy, the elimination of excessive regulation, the need to secure better value for the expenditure of Medicare dollars, the potential savings for beneficiaries and taxpayers, and the normative rationale for expanding patients' personal freedom in their choice and care and coverage. These reasons are still valid; in fact, even more so today.

Though America is politically polarized, Medicare's multiple problems—budgetary and programmatic—are of such a magnitude that Congress will be forced to come together and act, sooner or later. Medicare's rapidly growing enrollment, driven by millions of retiring baby boomers, will make unprecedented demands on the America's health care delivery systems. The traditional Medicare program, which is an outdated fee-for-service system of controlled prices, is governed in meticulous detail by a highly centralized bureaucracy that is often inflexible and sluggish in meeting new demands. The expansion of rapidly advancing medical technology, driven by dynamic biomedical research, benefits millions of Americans, but it also imposes ever larger costs on both beneficiaries and taxpayers alike. The perennial Medicare policy problem is not merely financing the cost of medical care but also securing the best value for those health care dollars, efficiently delivering better care at lower cost, and improving the health and the lives of millions of senior and disabled citizens who depend on the program.

The best way to achieve those goals is by harnessing the power of patient choice and genuine market competition. The best mechanism to harness that market power is through defined contribution (premium support) financing. Today, the great advantage for Washington's policymakers is that they have a solid record of experience in the performance of the Medicare Advantage program, the success of Medicare Part D in the competitive delivery of prescription drugs, and the stable continuity of the Federal Employees Health Benefits Program. Over decades, through trial and error, these programs have accumulated an impressive body of best practices.

Washington policymakers today can also tap into the rich body of policy work generated by the National Bipartisan Commission on the Future of Medicare as well as the independent work of a diverse group of analysts from the American Enterprise Institute, the Brookings Institution, the Heritage Foundation, and the Progressive Policy Institute. It is past time to revive what the *New York Times* editors once hailed as "the Medicare consensus."

• •

ROBERT EMMET MOFFIT, PhD, is a Senior Fellow in Domestic Policy Studies at the Heritage Foundation and served as Deputy Assistant Secretary for Legislation at the US Department of Health and Human Services during the Reagan administration.

NOTES

1. *New York Times*, "The New Consensus on Medicare," December 11, 1996. The referenced proposal was influenced by the research work of the Heritage Foundation on the viability of a defined contribution, premium support program. For the Heritage analysts, including the author, the financing and the light and flexible regulatory regime of the Federal Employees Health Benefits Program (FEHBP) was the preferred model for comprehensive reform. (Though it's worth noting, the model provided a template for key financing and regulatory changes to the Medicare program rather than a government-run structure to be adopted nationwide.)

2. "National Bipartisan Commission on the Future of Medicare," Library of Congress Web Archives, accessed November 20, 2021, https://www.loc.gov/item /lcwaN0003456.

3. The term "premium support" was coined by economists Henry Aaron and Robert Reischauer. See Henry J. Aaron and Robert D. Reischauer, "The Medicare Reform Debate: What Is the Next Step?," *Health Affairs* 14, no. 4 (Winter 1995): 8–30, https://www.healthaffairs.org/doi/abs/10.1377/hlthaff.14.4.8.

4. Sen. Ron Wyden (D-OR), "Wyden and Ryan Advance Bipartisan Plan to Strengthen Medicare and Expand Health Care Choices for All," December 15, 2011, https://www.wyden.senate.gov/news/press-releases/wyden-and-ryan-advance -bipartisan-plan-to-strengthen-medicare-and-expand-health-care-choices-for-all.

5. Boards of Trustees of the Federal Hospital Insurance and the Supplementary Medical Insurance Trust Funds, *2022 Annual Report of the Boards of Trustees*

(Washington, DC: Centers for Medicare and Medicaid Services, June 2, 2022), 6, https://www.cms.gov/files/document/2022-medicare-trustees-report.pdf. Hereafter cited as *2022 Medicare Trustees Report*

6. *2022 Medicare Trustees Report*, 6.

7. *2022 Medicare Trustees Report*, 27.

8. *2022 Medicare Trustees Report*, 8.

9. For the history of private plan participation in Medicare, see Thomas G. McGuire, Joseph P. Newhouse, and Anna D. Sinaiko, "An Economic History of Medicare Part C," *Milbank Quarterly* 89, no. 2 (June 2011): 289–332, https://onlinelibrary.wiley.com/doi/10.1111/j.1468-0009.2011.00629.x.

10. *2022 Medicare Trustees Report*, 67. That is also why a number of policy analysts have been proposing, among other specific measures, raising the normal age of Medicare eligibility and tracking future eligibility to increases in life expectancy. More importantly, it is a reason to revisit Medicare's outdated structure and introduce changes that would not only slow the growth of Medicare spending but secure higher quality care for future Medicare beneficiaries.

11. *2022 Medicare Trustees Report*, 93, table III.C5.

12. *2022 Medicare Trustees Report*, 38.

13. *2022 Medicare Trustees Report*, 101, table III.C10.

14. *2022 Medicare Trustees Report*, 40.

15. *2022 Medicare Trustees Report*, 41, table II.F3.

16. *2022 Medicare Trustees Report*, 9.

17. "A growing debt burden could increase the risk of a fiscal crisis and high inflation as well as undermine confidence in the US dollar, making it more costly to finance public and private activity in international markets." Congressional Budget Office, *The 2021 Long-Term Budget Outlook* (Washington, DC: Congressional Budget Office, March 2021), 1, https://www.cbo.gov/publication/57038.

18. *2022 Medicare Trustees Report*, 209.

19. *2022 Medicare Trustees Report*, 208, table V.F2.

20. See Robert E. Moffit, "Total Control: The House Democrats' Single Payer Health Care Prescription," Backgrounder no. 3423 (Washington, DC: The Heritage Foundation, July 19, 2019), https://www.heritage.org/sites/default/files/2019-07/BG3423.pdf.

21. Nina Owcharenko Shaefer and Robert E. Moffit, "The Public Option: Single Payer on the Installment Plan," Backgrounder, no. 3462 (Washington, DC: The Heritage Foundation, February 4, 2020), https://www.heritage.org/sites/default/files/2020-02/BG3462_0.pdf.

22. For an account of the price transparency initiatives, see Robert E. Moffit, "America Heads Closer to Medical Price Transparency," *The Hill*, November 2, 2020, https://thehill.com/opinion/healthcare/523979-america-heads-closer-to-medical-price-transparency-with-new-rule. On federal waivers, see Doug Badger, "How Health Care Premiums Are Declining in States that Seek Relief from Obamacare Mandates," Issue Brief no. 4990 (Washington, DC: The Heritage Foundation, August 13, 2019), https://www.heritage.org/sites/default/files/2019-08/IB4990.pdf.

23. *2022 Medicare Trustees Report*, 157, table IV.C1. In previous reports, federal actuaries generally underestimated the pace of Medicare Advantage enrollment. Doubtless the affordability of the Medicare Advantage health plans contributed to this rapid enrollment growth. See Centers for Medicare and Medicaid Services (CMS), "Trump Administration Announces Historically Low Medicare Advantage Premiums and New Payment Model to Make Insulin Affordable Again for Seniors," September 24, 2020, https://www.cms.gov/newsroom/press-releases/trump -administration-announces-historically-low-medicare-advantage-premiums-and -new-payment-model. Hereafter cited as CMS, "Trump Administration Announces Historically Low Medicare Advantage Premiums."

24. Analysts at the Heritage Foundation proposed the FEHBP as the model for reform, and the leaders of the commission agreed to advance that proposal. See Stuart M. Butler and Robert E. Moffit, "The FEHBP as a Model for a New Medicare Program," *Health Affairs* 14, no. 4 (Winter 1995): 47–61, https://www.healthaffairs .org/doi/abs/10.1377/hlthaff.14.4.47.

25. While the contributors to this volume largely embrace a full-scale defined contribution ("premium support") approach, Medicare inspires other major policy alternatives. For example, a group of scholars assembled by the Brookings Institution have focused on reforming Medicare Advantage's competitive bidding process. See Steven Lieberman, Loren Adler, Erin Trish, Joseph Antos, John Bertko, and Paul Ginsburg, "A Proposal to Enhance Competition and Reform Bidding in the Medicare Advantage Program," USC-Brookings Schaeffer Initiative for Health Policy, May 2018, https://www.brookings.edu/wp-content/uploads /2018/05/ma-bidding-paper.pdf. Impressed with Medicare Advantage's perfor-mance, some analysts favor "Medicare Advantage for All"; see Avik Roy, "Medicare Advantage: A Platform for Affordable Health Reform," Foundation for Research on Equal Opportunity, April, 18, 2019, https://freopp.org/medicare-advantage-a -platform-for-affordable-health-reform-fbe31bf444f3, and Billy Wynne, "The Bipartisan 'Single Payer' Solution: Medicare Advantage Premium Support for All," *Health Affairs Blog*, May 11, 2017, https://www.healthaffairs.org/do/10.1377 /hblog20170511.060017/full. Others propose using Medicare fee-for-service as a model for a national "single payer" health insurance system, even if it means repeal of the existing Medicare program, including Medicare Advantage. See, for example, Steffie Woolhander and David Himmelstein, "Single-Payer Reform—'Medicare for All,'" *Journal of the American Medical Association* 321, no. 24 (2019): 2399–2400, https://jamanetwork.com/journals/jama/article-abstract/2735406.

26. CMS, "Trump Administration Announces Historically Low Medicare Advantage Premiums."

27. Based on previous experience, there is reason to believe that more direct competition between private plans and traditional Medicare could improve the performance of the traditional program. In discussing the penetration of Medicare Advantage (MA) in certain counties, Joseph Newhouse and Thomas G. McGuire observe, "The available measures, while limited, suggest that, on average, MA plans offer care of equal or higher quality for less cost than traditional

Medicare (TM). In counties, greater MA penetration appears to improve TM's performance." See Joseph P. Newhouse and Thomas G. McGuire, "How Successful is Medicare Advantage," *Milbank Quarterly* 92, no. 2 (June 2014): 351–94, https://www.milbank.org/quarterly/articles/how-successful-is-medicare-advantage.

28. Bipartisan Policy Center, "Domenici-Rivlin Protect Medicare Act," BipartisanPolicy.org, released November 1, 2011, 3, https://bipartisanpolicy.org/download/?file=/wp-content/uploads/2019/03/Domenici-Rivlin-Protect-Medicare-Act-Backgrounder_0.pdf.

29. CMS, "Trump Administration Announces Historically Low Medicare Advantage Premiums."

PART I

THE CHALLENGE OF MEDICARE REFORM

Created in 1965, Medicare—the government program created to provide health coverage for America's seniors—faces significant challenges. Its traditional coverage model fails to achieve a core goal of health insurance: protecting enrollees against the financial risk of catastrophic illness. In 2028, given what we know today, a key part of the program will not be able to pay for all the promised hospital benefits. Meanwhile, the rapid rise in Medicare spending imposes large financial burdens on beneficiaries and taxpayers alike.

University of Pennsylvania economist Mark V. Pauly, PhD, observes that policymakers have been warned of Medicare's financial and structural challenges for decades, but it's been difficult to enact major structural reforms (chapter 2). Almost all policy responses (whether benefit expansion or cost cutting) made reforms within or additions to the current structure. Such options fall short of the challenge policymakers face today. Pauly finds promise for positive change in an alternative approach that seeks first to improve seniors' experience with Medicare by harnessing the power of competition in ways that also secure better financial value.

Such realities demand policymakers' attention, however, argues former Medicare trustee Charles P. Blahous, PhD, who outlines Medicare's emerging financial crisis and the sobering responsibilities that policymakers face in meeting this challenge (chapter 3).

Why Medicare Reform Has Been Hard

A Public Choice Perspective

The Medicare program, political experts tell us, is one of the most popular federal government programs, if not the most popular. So much so that any attempt to reform it runs the risk of electrocuting the change agents on the "third rail of politics."[1] Not only that, but a number of political entrepreneurs have borrowed the Medicare brand name (though not always its substance) to propose schemes for insurance for the rest of the US population.[2] But experts (sometimes the same ones) also tell us that Medicare is becoming fiscally unsustainable in its current form and needs some radical surgery, ideally before (and surely after) crashing into a financing wall.[3]

An important question I consider in this chapter is whether a majority of voters are likely to support some policy action that would reduce Medicare spending levels or growth. It should be noted, however, that unlike those who might advocate cutting Medicare spending primarily for budgetary reasons, the authors in this book emphasize the value of injecting stronger doses of consumer choice and competition into the Medicare program, potentially improving benefits and increasing the efficiency of the program's financing and delivery of care, and thus, securing, as a byproduct of these reforms, a slowdown in future spending growth.

In a democracy, public policy is not supposed to be up to elites or experts. Instead, voters express their preferences by choosing representatives who represent their views. Those views, however, are often divergent across voters depending both on their preferences and the tax structure for financing the cost of any policy change.

So what do different voters think about Medicare? Why is this almost 60-year-old program so allegedly revered and so evidently resistant thus far to explicit alteration? Some citizen misperception is always to be expected of any government activity, but such a stable history suggests that this arrangement provides more benefit than alternatives, not just to the representatives of the people but to at least enough of the people themselves in a majoritarian democracy.

In this chapter, I take an explicit "public choice" perspective that begins with those citizen preferences (for voters of different ages, incomes, and ideologies) for benefits in old age and the costs they must in some way bear.[4] I try to identify the sources of political popularity and stasis, and then I consider whether there might be alterations to the program that could generate enough additional net benefit for enough of the right kinds of voters to shift political choices by their representatives to ones that will avoid the expert-forecasted clash and crash described above. I will try to avoid value judgements (my own or anyone else's) about the merit of these changes.

Some General Observations: What Is the "Medicare Program"?

The legislation first enacted in 1965 to set up the Medicare health insurance program for the elderly (later extended to those with kidney failure and the disabled) has stood the test of time. Many of the original features of that program are still there. Some of the tail fins are gone, but the governmentally managed fee-for-service chassis and the 1960s model financing engine remain in place.

The biggest change, discussed in much of this book, is the addition of another option to that traditional Medicare model for those who want to choose it: a large number of privately administered Medicare Advantage plans with modestly different provider payment arrangements, benefit structures, and care management options. In my view, this makes today's Medicare Advantage a risk-adjusted "voucher" program with the dollar amount of the voucher determined by the cost of original Medicare. Premium support models differ formally from this model only in terms of how the voucher value is set. However, they differ politically because the original Medicare program would then no longer be guaranteed to have a premium linked to the value of the voucher with a zero additional premium (compared to other plans). One way to phrase the voter choice question in a concrete way is this: Could movement away from the current voucher arrangement linked to original Medicare get majority support?

Qualified health insurance under the traditional program is subsidized at about 90 percent for inpatient coverage (Part A) for persons with very low incomes. The optional parts of the program (Parts B and D) are subsidized at about 75 percent on top of beneficiary premiums that are means tested. All benefits are made available in the same amount to very wealthy people as to middle-class people; hence, redistribution based on benefits design and eligibility is not an apparent primary effect of the program. (However, there can still be a lot of redistribution going on, and the propensity of higher-income people to live longer and use more expensive care may further temper any redistribution.)[5] All Medicare Advantage plans must offer a specified set of benefits but can add additional benefits (at additional premiums to cover in full any additional costs if necessary). Private voluntary coverage (Medigap), lightly regulated, can be purchased to cover the cost sharing in the traditional public plan.

What is the nature of the benefits from this set of health insurance options? Health insurance of any type for this population is primarily a private good in that the value of both the health care it pays for and the reduction in financial risk it furnishes are obtained by insureds in the program and their families. There is in theory some external benefit to those not protected from coverage of care for contagious disease, but that value is minimal in the Medicare population (at least before coronavirus). More seriously, there are also, in theory, external benefits to family members and others who might otherwise be concerned about failure of their elders to use effective care or have adequate protection against illness-related financial risk.[6] The size of this consumption externality benefit or its distribution across the population are not matters of speculation. Who knows how much grandchildren would be willing to pay to make sure their grandparents have health insurance after the age of 65?

Who Gains and Who Loses?

The core premise of the public choice approach is that people choose political actions (voting, campaign contributions, canvassing) that might affect public programs by viewing those programs as any other commodity: on balance (taking any changes in taxes and any changes in benefits into account), will I be better off with one outcome compared to another? In this confusing mix of politics with representative government, people do not usually choose individual programs one at a time (as through a referendum); instead, they vote for one candidate over another based on their expected net benefit from the package of actions proposed or supported by each candidate. Here I will ignore the packaging or vote-trading aspects of multiple public programs to focus on Medicare. Realism requires that we add political ideology (whatever that may mean) as a finger on the scale, and a positive view of mankind requires that we assume that individuals may place positive values of the benefits of some actions to others than themselves for altruistic or ethical motives.

The simplest public choice model imagines that we can know the distribution of expected net benefits from the Medicare program over the voting-age population, as well as the propensity of different groups to vote. It then concludes that the collectively chosen option will be the one preferred by a majority of voters to any other option. If we can array the public good along a single scale (like cost or generosity of coverage), the model postulates that the outcome will usually be the one preferred by the person whose preferred option is the median (plus one) of all preferred options of all voters. The reason is that the option preferred by the "median person" can defeat any other option if voting takes place in a binary way. This model then implies that any proposal to reduce spending on that program will fail if it is not supported by the median voter.[7]

This model, like all models, permits exceptions when people cannot array options along the same scale (for example, if some people "most prefer" high spending but then next prefer zero spending) or if voting takes place in some other way.[8] However, it has served as a sturdy foundation to explain variation in the levels of public goods chosen in different communities or in the country at different points in time, so it is the one we will try here.

Down in the Weeds: Who Gains and Who Loses from Medicare?

There are three steps to the analysis of who gains and who loses from Medicare, and they get complicated fairly quickly. Let us think of the choice between two alternatives, today's Medicare program and some "reformed" alternative with lower spending and lower value of benefits. (I explore later why such an alternative will need to be considered.) There is no necessary reason that the value of benefits falls by the full amount of the dollar reduction in spending; the current level of spending may exceed the level at which the marginal benefit from that spending to actual or potential recipients exceeds its marginal cost. However, initially we will assume that the dollar value of reduction in well-being is equal to the dollar value of the spending reduction over the time period the person expected to receive Medicare benefits. Then we also need to know what is the reduction in tax cost to the person from now until the end of their lifetime.

Think of a worker currently age 50 who expects to retire and go on Medicare (Parts A, B, and D) in 15 years and then (on average) have 20 years more of life during which she receives a Medicare insurance plan that is worth about $17,000 a year—or an expected and discounted $351,000 over the person's expected lifetime after retiring at 65. (These are approximately realistic numbers for lifetime Medicare benefits, based on Kolasi and Steuerle 2020).[9] Suppose some new policy (premium support or some other), could reduce this spending by 1 percent, or $3,510, for this person and all others of the same age. That would amount to a reduction of $1,580 in the dollar value of Part A spending and a reduction of $1,930 in the value of all the other parts of Medicare using the current approximate 45 percent to 55 percent split.

Would this person gain more in reduced taxes than lose from this reduction in benefits? The answer depends primarily (ignoring possible changes in premiums) on the connection between any Medicare spending reduction and the person's future taxes. Here we assume that reductions in Part A spending translate into pro rata 1 percent reductions in the Medicare payroll tax (both worker and employer shares), while spending reduction in the other parts of Medicare reduce the person's income tax by 1 percent (whatever that tax will be).

Assume that this person has the $56,000 average income used in the Kolasi and Steurle example. Take first the case of all parts of Medicare other than Part A, which are financed by general revenue taxation. Taxes pay for 75 percent of the current approximately $440 billion per year cost of those benefits (or $330 billion) and that $330 billion is about 20 percent of total income tax collections of $1.6 trillion; we assume this share will continue for 15 years. For our assumed worker with the average income of a full-time worker of $56,000 a year, income tax would be $4,280 per year (according to one online federal tax calculator),[10] so the tax reduction from the 1 percent spending cut would be 0.2 percent of this. At the end of this long string of calculations we conclude that the person would save about $8.50 a year in income taxes or $130 over 15 years of remaining working life; this saving is much less than the loss in benefits and so this voter would disfavor the spending cut to Parts B and D.

Part A is financed by an earmarked payroll tax at 2.9 percent. How would a 1 percent cut in Part A spending affect our voter's taxes? If the payroll tax rate were changed, the person would save nothing in taxes. Instead, the primary benefit would be to extend the life of the trust fund until it hits a zero balance from the current anticipated data of 2024 by a few years. When the trust fund hits a zero balance, something will have to change. Working only within the Part A framework, we would say that either benefits would have to be cut or payroll taxes raised. If we assume the latter would happen, the 1 percent Part A spending reduction would postpone the time at which payroll taxes were raised and thus reduce total payroll taxes. The payroll tax on an income of $56,000 is about $1,600, so a 1 percent cut would be $16 per year, implying a total savings over 15 years of $240. This is higher than the income tax cut but still well below the dollar amount of lost benefits.

The conclusion therefore is that this person would lose from Medicare spending cuts over the retirement period. The size of the tax reductions is larger for younger people at the same income who will have more working years to pay taxes, but the net effect remains negative down to young ages. The median age of voters in the 2018 elections was about 52 years, so the great majority of older workers and younger workers with this income or less would oppose cuts. The median income is slightly below the average income used in the Kolasi-Steuerle example, suggesting added support to the conclusion that a 1 percent spending cut would fail to get majority approval. Specifically, almost all those currently on Medicare will oppose cuts, most of those (with below average or median incomes) at younger ages will also oppose, as will all low- (lifetime) income voters. High-income younger people would be the main opposition block, but they are unlikely to prevail. This simple thought experiment therefore suggests that change in Medicare will be rare (as has been true in the past) and will be difficult (in the future) unless some large negative impact of maintaining the current program spreads over many people at many incomes and ages. I consider the alternative reactions of reducing budget deficits or adding years of benefits to the Part A trust fund next.

Why Medicare Reform?

The demographics show that under current law most people (and most voters) would lose more dollars from Medicare's reduced spending than gain from the lower taxes they will expect to pay, and this runs into an iron law of arithmetic: future benefits greater than future payments cannot continue forever. Some way will have to be found to make up the difference. If spending is not reduced, either this social program will increase the federal debt, with whatever consequences flow from further kicking that can down the road, or someone will have to pay more in taxes.

This unlovely prospect has led many to worry that, regardless of how sacrosanct it is, Medicare must be reformed at some point in the future in a way that would lower the growth rate, and perhaps even the level, of spending per beneficiary, if only to bring the program back to some kind of fiscal balance—and these spending cuts could be arbitrary and without grace. One change in principle that could convert opposition to cuts into support for cuts would instead be some design that substantially improves the value of the benefit package relative to the amount spent on it.

This is not the place to advocate or even evaluate alternative care patterns that might wring more utility out of a given amount of Medicare spending across the board. If there is a better mousetrap, by all means beat a path to the door of the factory making it. However, recent history with attempts to improve Medicare through innovation in the original fee-for-service program have been very disappointing.

Offering competitive choice in the Medicare Advantage program has suggested more promise—as its plans are increasingly preferred to original Medicare—but the value of the gain from Medicare Advantage plans may not be large in absolute value even if it is enough to shift market share. Perhaps there might be somewhat less regulation and better tailoring of benefits to people with specific chronic conditions that would appeal to them. And the amount of waste to be cut cannot be unlimited.

Medicare premium support often has been advocated as a way of reducing the federal spending burden of Medicare over time, and one that will do a more graceful job of slowing spending than the price controls and ad hoc "annual productivity update" adjustments in original Medicare. Premium support can thus be a better way of avoiding the doomsday scenario. A common concern is that until the program actually hits some kind of fiscal wall, the prospect that it may do so (even with the common-sense caution that the carnage will be less severe if steps are taken in advance) may not be enough to change political preferences.

It does not seem at present that there is enough evidence to judge whether or when that might happen. Keeping track of the net benefit to that median or decisive set of voters will help us forecast the likelihood of change and the groups that need to be targeted with messaging about the need for and the benefit from change (compared to muddling through with the status quo for even longer).

Public Choice on the Day of Reckoning

Most of the discussion of Medicare's future focuses on actuarial data about projected spending and tax revenue relative to GDP (gross domestic product). The key metric here is the level and growth of spending per beneficiary and how much it can feasibly or plausibly grow over time. No one wants to forecast the impossible if there must eventually be a limit on spending for this program (and for Social Security) for the elderly.

Instead, the discussion asks what the decisive voter might choose in the face of a rising spending burden on the entire population for pensions and health insurance with some modest external benefits. That voter will surely be alerted to the consequences of burdening "future generations of grandchildren and great grandchildren" with heavy taxes or limited public services if those currently retired or near retirement do not agree to make do with less than under the status quo scenario. The alternative argument for spending cuts—that it will lengthen the time period in which Part A spending can be covered by the trust fund—is not likely to be attractive either, because this change only spreads the spending cuts over more years.

Economists know how to describe the potential adverse consequences of a growing lump of tax-financed spending on seniors from Medicare and Social Security (although they do not always agree on how likely or larger they are): that is, higher taxes and associated excess burden, tax distortion on work effort, investment and consumption, higher public debt relative to GDP with higher interest rates and interest payments, and displacement of other public goods of value. Logic dictates that if these adverse effects are large enough *and* impinge on the median voter, the majority-rule winner will be a proposal to reduce spending below what it would be with Medicare fee-for-service status quo and to go with some kind of Medicare premium support. It is hard to build macroeconomic disaster or public sector collapse into a rational voter model—so when and if this happens, all bets are off.

Right now, and for the foreseeable future, despite the impending zero balance in the Part A trust fund, it is hard to conclude that this decision-maker will support premium support that bites deeply into Medicare spending. Either the outlook and values of people on or near Medicare (in terms of their concern for the rest of the population and a realization that they did not pay for and are not entitled to the status quo benefits) will have to change, or the adverse macroeconomic consequences will have to get much worse and much more apparent.

Looking Ahead

A plausible, though simple, model of majoritarian democracy does not suggest that reform of Medicare based on arguments solely to lower its spending growth path is likely anytime soon. Most citizens, not just those who have retired but those in middle age, will expect to pay taxes that are much lower than the benefits they get. This happens both because the tax system is progressive and because some of the benefits are not fully funded by earmarked payroll taxes, so the cost of benefits will have to be paid by taxpayers in the distant future. There will have to be a more fundamental shift from the present state in the public sector's attention to balanced budget and adverse tax effects on incentives for policy on Medicare to change. We need stronger evidence to convince at least 50 percent plus one of our fellow citizens that this is the case. The authors of other chapters in this book focus on benefit changes and improvements that result incidentally in spending reductions; my analysis suggests this is a better path to try.

· ·

MARK V. PAULY is Professor Emeritus of Health Care Management at the Wharton School, University of Pennsylvania.

NOTES

1. Aaron Blake and Chris Cillizza, "Medicare: The New Third Rail of American Politics?," *Washington Post*, May 26, 2011, https://www.washingtonpost.com/blogs/the-fix/post/medicare-the-new-third-rail-of-american-politics/2011/05/25/AGzWLuBH_blog.html.

2. Sen. Bernie Sanders (D-VT), "Issues: Health Care as a Human Right—Medicare for All," accessed November 29, 2021, https://berniesanders.com/issues/medicare-for-all.

3. Boards of Trustees of the Federal Hospital Insurance and the Supplementary Medical Insurance Trust Funds, *2020 Annual Report of the Boards of Trustees* (Washington, DC: Centers for Medicare and Medicaid Service, April 22, 2020), https://www.cms.gov/files/document/2020-medicare-trustees-report.pdf.

4. James M. Buchanan and Gordon Tullock, *The Calculus of Consent: Logical Foundations of Constitutional Democracy* (Carmel, IN: The Liberty Fund, 1962).

5. Mark B. McClellan and Jonathan Skinner, "The Incidence of Medicare," NBER Working Paper no. 6013 (Cambridge, MA: National Bureau of Economic Research, April 1997), https://www.nber.org/papers/w6013.

6. Mark Pauly, *Medical Care at Public Expense: A Study in Applied Welfare Economics* (Westport, CT: Praeger, 1971).

7. Duncan Black, *The Theory of Committees and Elections* (Cambridge: Cambridge University Press, 1958).

8. Kenneth Arrow, *Social Choice and Individual Values* (New York: John Wiley, 1951).

9. Erald Kolasi and C. Eugene Steuerle, *Social Security & Medicare Lifetime Benefits & Taxes: 2020* (Washington, DC: Tax Policy Center of the Urban Institute and Brookings Institution, November 17, 2020), https://www.urban.org/sites /default/files/publication/103243/social-security-and-medicare-lifetime-benefits -and-taxes-2020_0.pdf.

10. "Federal Income Tax Calculator," SmartAsset.com, accessed November 29, 2021, https://smartasset.com/taxes/income-taxes.

Pursuing Medicare Reform in the Context of a Financing Crisis

Medicare faces a looming financing crisis, which has only grown more urgent due to the economic damage wrought by the COVID-19 pandemic. Federal lawmakers will have no choice but to act soon to shore up Medicare's solvency, whether by slowing the growth of program costs, raising eligibility ages, increasing taxes, or a combination of all three. All decisions about the future design and scope of Medicare will be made in the context of this overriding financial challenge.

Even before the pandemic hit, Medicare was heading into trouble. Medicare's hospital insurance (HI) program—the one part of Medicare that can experience a depletion of its financial resources—entered calendar year 2020 with a trust fund balance sufficient only to fund less than seven months' worth of benefit payments.[1] This meant that its near-term financial stability depended largely on whether incoming payroll tax revenues would be nearly sufficient by themselves to fund outgoing benefit payments. The Medicare trustees' report released in June 2022 projected that this delicate balancing act would be sustained only until 2028, at which point the hospital insurance program would become insolvent. Insolvency, in this context, means that the HI trust fund will not be able to provide all of the promised hospital benefits at the projected level of dedicated financing under current law.

Impending Medicare HI insolvency is a sizable enough problem by itself, but it actually represents less than half of the larger Medicare financing challenge. The greater part of Medicare, which covers physician services, prescription drugs, and all other benefits routed through its supplementary medical insurance (SMI) trust fund, faces an even more severe cost growth problem. Medicare SMI is statutorily constructed so that technically it cannot become insolvent; premium assessments on SMI beneficiaries, and contributions of federal general revenues, are automatically increased each year in the amounts necessary to fund benefit payments. However, the absence of insolvency within SMI doesn't mean that it lacks financing strains. It simply means that the pain of its uncontrolled cost growth is felt in different ways by different people (e.g., premium-paying beneficiaries and federal taxpayers).

The rising costs of Medicare SMI could well be considered the most daunting Medicare-related challenge facing lawmakers, greater even than Medicare HI's impending insolvency. The trustees had estimated that Medicare SMI would require $377 billion in general revenue funding in 2020 alone.[2] This draw on general government revenues exists above and beyond all other Medicare financing sources, including the payroll taxes collected for Medicare HI, and premiums paid by and on behalf of Medicare beneficiaries. Going forward, these pressures on the federal budget will only intensify (as illustrated in fig. 3.1). Medicare SMI costs are growing so rapidly that by 2035 they are projected to absorb a share of US gross domestic product (GDP) that is more than 50 percent larger than they do today.[3]

This cost growth will also drain the pocketbooks of Medicare's aged beneficiaries by reducing the effective purchasing power of their monthly Social Security checks. Under current law, average Medicare Part B and Part D premiums are projected to soar from 13 percent of the average Social Security benefit today to 19 percent by the end of the trustees' 75-year valuation window.[4]

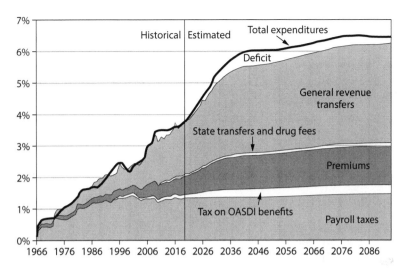

FIGURE 3.1. Medicare Costs and Revenue Sources as a Percentage of Gross Domestic Product. Projected Medicare obligations will swamp the federal budget. *Source*: Boards of Trustees of the Federal Hospital Insurance and Federal Supplementary Medical Insurance Trust Funds, *2020 Annual Report of the Boards of Trustees* (Washington, DC: Centers for Medicare and Medicaid Services, April 22, 2020), figure I.1, https://www.cms .gov/files/document/2020-medicare-trustees-report.pdf (prepandemic projections).

Sobering though these numbers are, they reflect a relatively optimistic take on Medicare's future. Specifically, they assume that certain ambitious cost-containment provisions of the 2010 Affordable Care Act (ACA) are successful and remain in force. The ACA instated gradual reductions in Medicare provider payment growth, which subtract roughly 1 percent each year from annual payment updates.[5] The compounding effects of these annual adjustments will widen an already large differential between Medicare and private insurance payment rates. For example, Medicare payment rates for inpatient hospital care are currently only about 60 percent of what they are under private insurance. The Office of the Actuary at the Centers for Medicare and Medicaid Services (CMS), the agency that administers the program, projects that due to the ACA, Medicare payment rates for inpatient hospital care will eventually decline to roughly 40 percent of what private insurance pays on average.[6]

No one knows the consequences of such a vast divergence between future Medicare and private payment rates, a situation that subjects program participants to tremendous uncertainty. For example, Medicare's actuaries have expressed concern that pushing Medicare provider payment rates so far below private insurance rates—which would also be well below providers' reported costs of operation—could result in "access and quality-of-care issues for Medicare beneficiaries."[7] This in turn could drive mounting political pressure to eventually repeal these provisions of the ACA. If that happens, Medicare costs will be even higher than current projections show, accelerating HI insolvency and requiring still greater sacrifices from beneficiaries and taxpayers. Fortunately, from the perspective of Medicare finances, if not from the perspective of providers, the ACA's payment adjustments have thus far been sustained.

Medicare's enormous financial challenge is made more urgent and immediate by the COVID-afflicted American economy. The downturn triggered by the pandemic affected Medicare finances in several ways, the most significant being a reduction in payroll tax collections. The Congressional Budget Office (CBO) indicated in 2022 that there were fewer than five months' worth of benefit payments in Medicare's HI trust fund.[8] Instead of indulging in fanciful debates about whether to expand Medicare, lower its age of eligibility, or, even more grandiosely, enact "Medicare for All" (the name commonly applied to current proposals to have the federal government provide comprehensive health insurance for all Americans), federal lawmakers will likely need to enact legislation merely to prevent the current Medicare program from becoming insolvent during the late 2020s.

Impact on Beneficiaries

This blizzard of data must not blind us to the reality that Medicare finances are not simply a matter of abstract lines plotted on graphs. There are real people behind all these numbers, and they suffer real hardship so long as Medicare finances remain uncorrected.

It's obvious that Medicare beneficiaries would suffer greatly if law-makers were ever to permit Medicare HI to become insolvent. Under federal law, if this were to happen, then payments to health providers would be suddenly interrupted, precipitating immediate disruptions of health care access. According to the Medicare trustees' latest projections, 10 percent of Medicare HI obligations would go unpaid in the year following trust fund depletion.[9] Such a sudden disruption of access to hospital care could have unimaginably severe health consequences for American seniors.

But far beyond the solvency of this one Medicare trust fund, Americans are generally made poorer by the larger federal policy failure to contain the growth of Medicare costs. Excess health price inflation, which is exacerbated by a wide range of US government policies, inevitably limits the quantity and quality of care that Americans can receive for every dollar they spend. Rising health costs place American households under worsening financial stress, irrespective of whether these costs are borne out of pocket, deducted from take-home wages, or reflected in tax burdens. The increasing share of federal spending absorbed by health programs gradually stifles government's ability to meet other national needs and to serve the public in other ways. Simply put, we are losing control of our financial future due to these health policy failures, both at the household level and at the government level.

A lasting solution to these problems requires that federal policies be reformed to slow the growth of Medicare costs specifically, and health care costs more generally. These objectives dovetail with widespread desire among the American public to sustain the Medicare program on which tens of millions have come to depend. The irony is that Medicare as we know it cannot be preserved unless it is significantly changed.

The Successes of Medicare Advantage

Amid the daunting numbers that have proliferated throughout annual Medicare trustees' reports in recent years, there have been pockets of good news—areas where Medicare has outperformed expectations. One of them is the Medicare Advantage (MA) program.

MA is a feature of Medicare through which beneficiaries can receive Medicare coverage from private insurance plans. Medicare pays a fixed amount to cover each beneficiary enrolled in an MA plan, which in turn provides the participating individual with Part A (hospital insurance) coverage, Part B (physician and other medical insurance) coverage, and often Part D (prescription drug) coverage as well, in addition to other benefits such as vision, hearing, and dental care.[10] Growing numbers of American seniors are concluding that the private health plans offering coverage under MA meet their needs more effectively than does traditional Medicare.

Medicare has offered private plan enrollment options since its inception, but the MA program as it operates today really took shape because of the 2003 Medicare Modernization Act (MMA).[11] When the 2003 MMA was passed, private plan enrollment in Medicare stood at just over 5 million, or roughly 13 percent of participants. After the enactment of the MMA, Medicare Advantage enrollment took off dramatically, surpassing 11 million, or 24 percent of participants, by the time the Congress debated the ACA in 2009 and 2010.[12]

Some analysts attributed the post-MMA increases in Medicare Advantage enrollment to Medicare's then paying MA plans a larger amount per beneficiary than was provided under traditional fee-for-service (FFS) Medicare.[13] The ACA's sponsors sought to end this imbalance by enacting reductions, beginning in 2012, in MA benchmark payments so that MA payments per capita would no longer exceed the amounts spent in the publicly administered Medicare FFS program.

Government forecasters expected that once MA plans' perceived subsidy advantage was eliminated, the plans would become less attractive and enrollment would therefore decline. Specifically, the 2010 Medicare trustees' report, published immediately after the ACA's enactment, anticipated that MA enrollment would decline from a peak of about 12 million in 2012 (24 percent of Medicare beneficiaries) to about 8 million in 2020 (13 percent of beneficiaries).[14]

This expected decline in MA enrollment never happened. Despite the ACA's cuts in federal payments to MA plans, enrollment continued to grow dramatically. In 2020 it stood at roughly 25 million, or approximately 40 percent of all Medicare beneficiaries—over three times the enrollment projected in the wake of the ACA (as shown in fig. 3.2).[15] Medicare beneficiaries have increasingly voted with their feet and are walking away from traditional Medicare as they find that for the same amount of money, private plans under MA are better able to meet their coverage needs.

Annual Medicare trustees' reports throughout the last decade have repeatedly expressed surprise over MA plans' rising popularity. The 2010 trustees' report, released immediately after the ACA, noted that "the Affordable Care Act reduces Medicare payments to private plans" and predicted that this would "result in less-generous plan benefit packages and/or higher premiums." Consequently, "enrollment in MA plans is expected to decline in the future, both in number and as a percent of total beneficiaries."[16] But just four years later, the trustees' 2014 report noted, "the Trustees previously estimated that plan enrollment would decrease, starting in 2011, as a result of the benchmark and rebate changes in the Affordable Care Act." Instead, "between 2004 and 2013,

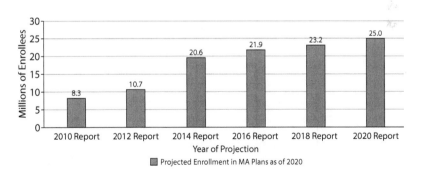

FIGURE 3.2. Medicare Advantage Enrollment Repeatedly Surpassing Trustees' Projections. *Source*: Boards of Trustees of the Federal Hospital Insurance and Federal Supplementary Medical Insurance Trust Funds, *2020 Annual Report of the Boards of Trustees* (Washington, DC: Centers for Medicare and Medicaid Services, April 22, 2020), 150, table IV.C1, https://www.cms.gov/files/document/2020-medicare-trustees-report.pdf.

private plan enrollment grew by 9.5 million or 176 percent, which compares to growth in the overall Medicare population of 25 percent for the same period."[17] Since that 2014 report, enrollment in MA has only continued to exceed prior trustees' projections. MA's enrollment in 2021 of nearly 28 million was substantially greater than the 2014 report's revised projection of 20.6 million.[18]

Annual trustees' reports offer various explanations for Medicare Advantage enrollments surpassing previous estimates, but while explanations have evolved and projections have been updated, the phenomenon of higher-than-projected numbers has persisted with remarkable consistency. The inescapable conclusion is that Medicare Advantage has simply been able to offer more value than government experts had forecast. As a result, as the 2014 trustees' report notes, "the effect of the ACA benchmark reductions [MA payment rate on MA enrollment] was less than previously assumed."[19] Evidence of MA's unexpected performance is scattered throughout the trustees' reports, for example in 2013 it states, "in this year's report, the Medicare Advantage plan bid assumptions were lowered to reflect recent data suggesting that certain provisions of the Affordable Care Act will reduce growth in these costs by more than was previously projected."[20]

This all raises the question as to whether the surprising success of Medicare Advantage in cutting costs has been achieved by shifting burdens to beneficiaries. Thus far, this does not appear to be the case. First, if it were, it's doubtful that so many more Medicare beneficiaries would voluntarily choose to enroll in MA. Other data support the view that MA is providing real value to beneficiaries. The Kaiser Family Foundation finds that "premiums paid by Medicare Advantage enrollees have slowly declined since 2015," even as premiums in traditional Medicare have steadily grown.[21] Researchers writing in the *American Journal of Managed Care* also find that "although MA payment cuts were expected to reduce the attractiveness of the MA program to both plans and enrollees, the program's enrollment grew steadily from 2009 to 2017. Over this period, plans reduced their costs for providing Part A and Part B benefits to their enrollees, thereby preserving room for rebates. Our findings show that plans made such cost reductions without significantly affecting enrollees' access to or affordability of care compared with TM [traditional Medicare] beneficiaries."[22]

While Medicare as a whole faces mounting challenges, the market competition occurring within Medicare Advantage among private health plans is producing results that have repeatedly surpassed government forecasters' expectations. As policymakers wrestle with the difficult choices for stabilizing Medicare, they will need to derive lessons from where Medicare is working well, as much as from those aspects of Medicare that need to change.

Looking Ahead

The primary focus here is on the financial challenges facing Medicare, which will require lawmakers to enact legislation in the near-term to preserve Medicare HI solvency and, at least at some point, to slow the growth of broader program costs. Lawmakers will need to make a number of inherently subjective value judgements in the course of fulfilling this responsibility. However, a wide range of philosophical preferences would be served by policy choices that render Medicare's financial challenges more manageable.

Medicare beneficiaries and federal taxpayers are benefiting from the efficiencies achieved through the competitive processes in Medicare Advantage. To the extent that MA has presented financial incentives to competing health insurers, these insurers have responded by finding ways to lower their costs, while reducing premiums and out-of-pocket expenses facing program beneficiaries. Individual participants have also responded to these incentives by enrolling in MA plans in escalating numbers. Trends to date suggest that additional savings might be achieved by making the financial incentives facing participants and insurance providers more robust and transparent, as well as by increasing the flexibility afforded to competing health insurers, specifically by widening their latitude to offer insurance coverage of varying design.

In recent decades, bipartisan proposals to constrain Medicare cost growth while limiting adverse impacts on beneficiaries have typically included some variant of a defined contribution or premium support financing model. Under a premium support approach, Medicare would provide a specified amount of funding for each individual beneficiary, irrespective of whether the individual enrolls in traditional Medicare FFS or a private plan.[23] Among the notable premium support proposals debated in recent decades are those developed by the Breaux-Thomas Medicare Commission in 1999, by Rep. Paul Ryan (R-WI) and Sen. Ron Wyden (D-OR) in 2011, and by the Bipartisan Policy Center (Rivlin-Domenici). The Congressional Budget Office has projected that reforms based on premium support could slow the growth of Medicare costs considerably, although the amount saved would vary widely depending on how payment levels are set as a function of private insurer bids, and on whether current participants in traditional Medicare are moved into the premium support system or grandfathered into their current form of coverage.[24]

Regardless of the policy direction lawmakers choose, repairing Medicare finances will require tough choices that even the most well-designed reforms cannot wholly eliminate. This is because Medicare, as a program for the aged, is being buffeted by powerful demographic forces. As Americans live longer lives, and as more members of the historically large baby boom generation enter the ranks of retired beneficiaries, we cannot avoid the necessity of striking difficult balances between how much support beneficiaries receive during their retirement years, how many years of life these benefits cover, and how high tax burdens should be set. Consider, for example, that baby boomer retirements are driving growth in Social Security costs that far exceed growth in US economic output, increasing from 4.2 percent of GDP at the start of 2008 to a projected 5.9 percent of GDP in the mid-2030s, even without Social Security outlays being affected nearly as much as Medicare's by the rising cost of health care.[25] Hence, even if reforms succeeded perfectly in taming excess health cost inflation, rising

Medicare costs would still need to be managed and ameliorated in other ways.

In addition, as is often noted in financial markets, "past performance is no guarantee of future results." The fact that MA has managed to produce so many efficiency gains over the past decade does not necessarily mean it will continue to do so at the same rate going forward. Waste that has already been wrung out of the system cannot be re-eliminated. Lawmakers therefore cannot take it for granted that expanding MA would empower private insurers to generate cost savings even more successfully than they have done during the past several years. In addition, the potential for savings would depend, in part, on the scope, design, and details of any such expansion. Still, any cost savings achieved relative to current projections would somewhat relax the necessity of making other difficult choices to stabilize Medicare finances.

Medicare currently faces a future of unaffordable cost growth and a looming financial shortfall, which is quickly becoming more urgent due to the economy being weakened by COVID-19. To repair program finances with least harm to beneficiaries, lawmakers will need to find ways to build upon those parts of Medicare that are providing the greatest value for the money.

• •

CHARLES P. BLAHOUS, PhD, was a public trustee for Social Security and Medicare from 2010 through 2015. He currently holds the J. Fish and Lillian F. Smith Chair at the Mercatus Center at George Mason University and is a Visiting Fellow at the Hoover Institution at Stanford University.

NOTES

1. Boards of Trustees of the Federal Hospital Insurance and the Supplementary Medical Insurance Trust Funds, *2020 Annual Report of the Boards of Trustees* (Washington, DC: Centers for Medicare and Medicaid Services, April 22, 2020), 57, table III.B6, https://www.cms.gov/files/document/2020-medicare-trustees-report.pdf. Hereafter cited as *2020 Medicare Trustees Report*.

2. Social Security and Medicare Boards of Trustees, *Status of the Social Security and Medicare Programs: A Summary of the 2020 Annual Reports* (Baltimore: Social

Security Office of the Chief Actuary, 2020), 8, https://www.ssa.gov/OACT/TRSUM/tr20summary.pdf.

3. Boards of Trustees of the Federal Hospital Insurance and the Supplementary Medical Insurance Trust Funds, *2022 Annual Report of the Boards of Trustees* (Washington, DC: Centers for Medicare and Medicaid Services, June 2, 2022), 179, table V.B2, https://www.cms.gov/files/document/2022-medicare-trustees-report.pdf. Hereafter cited as *2022 Medicare Trustees Report*.

4. *2022 Medicare Trustees Report*, 39.

5. *2020 Medicare Trustees Report*, 4.

6. John D. Shatto and M. Kent Clemens, *Projected Medicare Expenditures under an Illustrative Scenario with Alternative Payment Updates to Medicare Providers* (Baltimore: Centers for Medicare and Medicaid, Office of the Actuary, June 2, 2022), 5, fig. 1, https://www.cms.gov/files/document/illustrative-alternative-scenario-2022.pdf.

7. Shatto and Clemens, 7.

8. Congressional Budget Office, *10-Year Trust Fund Projections: May 2022*, table 3, https://www.cbo.gov/data/budget-economic-data#5.

9. Social Security and Medicare Boards of Trustees, *Status of the Social Security and Medicare Programs: A Summary of the 2022 Annual Reports* (Baltimore: Social Security Office of the Chief Actuary, 2022), 4, https://www.ssa.gov/OACT/TRSUM/tr22summary.pdf.

10. "How Do Medicare Advantage Plans Work?," Medicare.gov, accessed October 12, 2021, https://www.medicare.gov/sign-up-change-plans/types-of-medicare-health-plans/medicare-advantage-plans/how-do-medicare-advantage-plans-work.

11. Yash Patel and Stuart Guterman, *The Evolution of Private Plans in Medicare* (New York: The Commonwealth Fund, December 8, 2017), 6–7, https://www.commonwealthfund.org/publications/issue-briefs/2017/dec/evolution-private-plans-medicare.

12. Boards of Trustees of the Federal Hospital Insurance and the Supplementary Medical Insurance Trust Funds, *2010 Annual Report of the Boards of Trustees* (Washington, DC: Centers for Medicare and Medicaid Services, August, 5, 2010), 198, table IV.C1, https://www.cms.gov/Research-Statistics-Data-and-Systems/Statistics-Trends-and-Reports/ReportsTrustFunds/Downloads/TR2010.pdf. Hereafter, *2010 Medicare Trustees Report*.

13. Robert Berenson and Melissa Goldstein, "Will Medicare Wither on the Vine? How Congress Has Advantaged Medicare Advantage—And What's a Level Playing Field Anyway?," *Saint Louis University Journal of Health Law & Policy* 1, no. 1 (2007): 7–8.

14. *2010 Medicare Trustees Report*, 198, table IV.C1.

15. *2022 Medicare Trustees Report*, 157, table IV.C1.

16. *2010 Medicare Trustees Report*, 49.

17. Boards of Trustees of the Federal Hospital Insurance and the Supplementary Medical Insurance Trust Funds, *2014 Annual Report of the Boards of Trustees*

(Washington, DC: Centers for Medicare and Medicaid Services, July 28, 2014), 161, https://www.cms.gov/Research-Statistics-Data-and-Systems/Statistics-Trends -and-Reports/ReportsTrustFunds/Downloads/TR2014.pdf. Hereafter cited as *2014 Medicare Trustees Report.*

18. *2014 Medicare Trustees Report*, 163, table IV.C1.

19. *2014 Medicare Trustees Report*, 162.

20. Boards of Trustees of the Federal Hospital Insurance and the Supplementary Medical Insurance Trust Funds, *2013 Annual Report of the Boards of Trustees* (Washington, DC: Centers for Medicare and Medicaid Services, May 31, 2013), 76, https://www.cms.gov/Research-Statistics-Data-and-Systems/Statistics-Trends -and-Reports/ReportsTrustFunds/Downloads/TR2013.pdf.

21. Gretchen Jacobson, Meredith Freed, Anthony Damico, and Tricia Neuman, "A Dozen Facts about Medicare Advantage in 2019," Kaiser Family Foundation, June 6, 2019, https://www.kff.org/medicare/issue-brief/a-dozen-facts-about -medicare-advantage-in-2019.

22. Laura Skopec, Joshua Aarons, and Stephen Zuckerman, "Did Medicare Advantage Payment Cuts Affect Beneficiary Access and Affordability?," *American Journal of Managed Care* 25, no. 9 (2019): e261. Another factor of note was the demonstration program initiated by the Obama administration to pay bonuses to plans with three- and three-and-one-half-star ratings, going beyond the bonuses authorized in the ACA for plans with quality ratings of four stars or more. The demonstration alleviated the effects of the ACA's payment cuts for certain plans. See Laura Skopec, Stephen Zuckerman, Eva Allen, and Joshua Aarons, *Why Did Medicare Advantage Enrollment Grow as Payment Pressure Increased? Examining the Role of Market and Demographic Changes* (Washington, DC: Urban Institute, April 24, 2019), https://www.urban.org/sites/default/files/publication/100152 /why_did_medicare_advantage_enrollment_grow_as_payment_pressure_increased _1.pdf.

23. MedPAC, *June 2017 Report to the Congress: Medicare and the Health Care Delivery System* (Washington, DC: Medicare Payment Advisory Commission, 2017), 75, https://www.medpac.gov/wp-content/uploads/import_data/scrape_files/docs /default-source/reports/jun17_reporttocongress_sec.pdf.

24. Congressional Budget Office, *A Premium Support System for Medicare*, October 2017, 6, table 1, https://www.cbo.gov/system/files/115th-congress-2017 -2018/reports/53077-premiumsupport.pdf.

25. "OASDI and HI Annual Income, Cost, and Balance as a Percentage of GDP, Calendar Years 1970–2095," in *2022 Annual Report of the Board of Trustees of the Federal Old-Age and Survivors Insurance and Federal Disability Insurance Trust Funds* (Washington, DC: Social Security Administration, 2022), table VI.G4, https://www .ssa.gov/OACT/TR/2022/VI_G2_OASDHI_GDP.html#200732.

PART II

MEDICARE ADVANTAGE
The Record and Opportunity

Medicare today consists of two main types of benefit delivery models: a system of competing private health plans (which includes Medicare Advantage) and a system in which government officials set fees for services offered (traditional Medicare)

This section examines the case-study lessons Medicare Advantage offers policymakers seeking to improve Medicare, finding it delivers greater value for beneficiaries while delivering benefits at competitive prices. This success is driven by the value it offers, as Christopher Pope, PhD, finds in his examination of the program's proven record of success for enrollees and taxpayers (chapter 4). As the program also has room to improve, John C. Goodman, PhD, suggests ways to build on its successes with additional consumer-friendly reforms (chapter 5).

Dr. Brian J. Miller, MD, and Gail R. Wilensky, PhD, argue that the successes of Medicare Advantage suggest that a promising first step in comprehensive Medicare reform is to leverage a quietly emerging reality: Medicare enrollees are self-selecting into Medicare Advantage rather than traditional Medicare (chapter 6). As the Medicare trustees reported in 2020, between 2010 and 2019 alone private plan enrollment grew by 96 percent, while the total Medicare population grew by 28 percent. Default enrollment of new beneficiaries into Medicare Advantage, rather than the traditional program, would help stabilize the overall program while supporting patient personal choices of plans and benefits.

How Medicare Advantage Secures Better Value for Seniors and Taxpayers

In Medicare, the federal program that serves senior and disabled citizens, there are two vastly different systems for financing and delivering comprehensive health insurance benefits. The traditional Medicare program, enacted in 1965, is a "single payer" program, where the government determines purchase terms for all medical services. Under Medicare Advantage (MA), a growing system of competing private health plans created in 2003, the government makes per capita contribution to a participating health plan chosen each year by Medicare beneficiaries.

Traditional Medicare has routinely paid fixed rates for each medical service that is provided to beneficiaries. This has made it highly susceptible to interest group lobbying over reimbursement, caused it to overpay for services that offer little value, while leaving uncovered cost-effective services for which billing codes had not been established.

Medicare Advantage plans offer better value to beneficiaries because they are paid up-front sums to deliver a comprehensive package of health care services to enrollees. This model creates incentives for plans to find lower-cost ways of obtaining medical services while also developing innovative ways to keep enrollees healthy and avoid costly hospitalizations.

Medicare Advantage plans cut costs by steering enrollees to networks of preferred providers, with which it has negotiated discounted rates. They also design benefits to encourage patients to first visit primary care practitioners and to receive medical procedures from outpatient facilities. Plans can target added care coordination services and preventive care at enrollees with chronic illnesses who are responsible for the bulk of the program's costs.

Medicare Advantage enrollees suffer fewer hospitalizations and readmissions than Medicare beneficiaries with equivalent medical risks who remain in the fee-for-service public option. Where policy changes have suddenly drawn more beneficiaries into Medicare Advantage, increased enrollment in these plans has been found to significantly reduce their mortality rate. Medicare beneficiaries who are enrolled in Medicare Advantage suffer fewer costly, painful, and ineffective medical procedures in their last few months of life and are more likely to receive appropriate palliative care.

Even after counting profits and administrative costs that are incurred, the cost at which Medicare Advantage plans bid to deliver the standard package of Medicare benefits averages 12 percent less than the expense incurred for beneficiaries with equivalent medical needs who remain in the traditional public option. Plans may use these savings to attract enrollees with enhanced benefits, typically including dental coverage, premium-free prescription drug coverage, and limits on out-of-pocket costs, for which enrollees would otherwise have needed to purchase costly supplemental insurance.

Flawed Attempts to Reform Fee-For-Service

Traditional Medicare providers may claim more money from the federal government if they order unhelpful diagnostic tests, perform unnecessary procedures, or make mistakes that must be corrected with follow-up appointments. In 2011, for example, the readmission of patients within 30 days following a hospitalization cost Medicare $24 billion—11 percent of its total spending on hospital care.[1]

To remedy these problems, Congress enacted a complex system of adjustments to provider fees in the 2015 Medicare Access and CHIP Reauthorization Act and Title III of the 2010 Affordable Care Act. Yet these amendments have complicated the practice of medicine without fundamentally changing the incentives to inflate costs and service volumes.[2]

By contrast, Medicare Advantage plans in each county receive an up-front monthly payment from the federal government for each Medicare beneficiary that opts to enroll in them. This payment is based on a combination of the per-beneficiary level of Medicare spending in the local area, the plan's bid as to its expected cost of delivering the standard package of Medicare benefits, and its score on a system of quality metrics.[3]

How Medicare Advantage Delivers Lower Care Costs

Medicare Advantage plans are responsible for purchasing health care services for beneficiaries, a requirement that gives the plans an incentive to find lower-cost ways of procuring medical services and develop ways of preventing expensive hospitalizations altogether.[4] Whereas every price and payment arrangement for tens of thousands of services under the traditional fee-for-service Medicare benefit is the subject of fierce political conflict and lobbying by medical providers, Medicare Advantage plans are operated privately and so can purchase services more selectively to get better value for money.[5]

The traditional fee-for-service Medicare benefit reimburses medical claims without consideration of whether more cost-effective alternatives are available. Because it verifies the legitimacy of less than 0.3 percent of 1.3 billion payments to providers that it makes every year, the fee-for-service Medicare program is therefore highly vulnerable to fraud.[6] The US Department of Health and Human Services estimated that 6.3 percent of claims reimbursed by Medicare in 2020 ought not to have been paid—costing taxpayers $26 billion.[7] By contrast, Medicare Advantage plans typically review the merits of medical claims before and after payment.

Though traditional Medicare is typically able to purchase hospital care at lower prices than employer-sponsored insurance, Medicare Advantage is still able to negotiate a better deal.[8] Medicare Advantage plans pay, on average, 30 percent less for durable medical equipment and diagnostic rates than the traditional fee-for-service Medicare program by purchasing products at commercially available rates rather than politically established prices.[9] By establishing networks of preferred providers, Medicare Advantage plans are able to pay physicians on average 3 percent less than fee-for-service Medicare for equivalent procedures.[10] They are able to pay hospitals 8 percent less per equivalent admission—even though MA enrollees admitted to hospital tend to be relatively sicker—because plans also save money by having less severely ill patients treated on an outpatient basis.[11]

Medicare beneficiaries enrolled in Medicare Advantage are 7 percent less likely to undergo surgery on an inpatient basis than other beneficiaries with equivalent medical risks but 25 percent more likely to receive outpatient surgery. Medicare Advantage enrollees make 22 percent fewer visits to specialists but only 3 percent fewer consultations with primary care physicians.[12]

Medicare Advantage's Focus on Preventative Care

Whereas Medicare's traditional payment arrangements reimburse providers of new and costlier ways of treating patients, regardless of whether they deliver better outcomes, Medicare Advantage's payment arrangement encourages the development of new methods of delivering medical care that save money. As most beneficiaries tend to remain enrolled in the same Medicare Advantage plans from year to year, insurers know that they are likely to be responsible for their medical costs as patients develop major illnesses in subsequent years and therefore have an incentive to invest in preventative care.[13]

Medicare Advantage plans benefit most from savings on diseases amenable to management by primary care (such as diabetes, chronic heart failure, or chronic obstructive pulmonary disease), which allows patients to avoid needless consultations with expensive specialists.[14] Enrollees of Medicare Advantage managed care plans who were at risk of breast cancer, diabetes, and cardiovascular disease are 5 percent to 20 percent more likely than other Medicare patients to receive appropriate tests.[15] Disabled Medicare beneficiaries with breast cancer who were enrolled in Medicare Advantage plans were diagnosed earlier and had higher survival rates than those who remained enrolled in traditional Medicare.[16]

Medicare beneficiaries enrolled in Medicare Advantage managed care plans were also 22 percent more likely to receive annual flu shots and pneumococcal vaccinations.[17] Indeed, concerns that a spike in seasonal flu cases would coincide with a winter wave of COVID-19 led UnitedHealthcare in 2020 to send its Medicare Advantage enrollees special flu kits that included a supply of the antiviral Tamiflu.[18]

Medicare Advantage's payment arrangements also allow plans to provide additional home care services to Medicare beneficiaries with chronic conditions to help them avoid hospitalizations. For instance, Humana-at-Home offers 24-7 support for house calls, additional maintenance visits to help proactively monitor chronic illnesses, and continuity-of-care services to assist with transitions back home following hospitalizations, which help prevent readmissions.[19] Medicare beneficiaries with diabetes who were enrolled in a Medicare Advantage special needs plan that offered preventive house calls, medication assistance, and post-hospitalization assistance visited physicians' offices 7 percent more than a control group that remained in traditional Medicare, but they spent 19 percent fewer days in hospital.[20]

Recent legislation and regulatory changes have made it easier for Medicare Advantage plans to offer additional nonmedical benefits targeted at enrollees with chronic conditions such as heart failure, rheumatoid arthritis, Alzheimer's, or Parkinson's disease. For instance, plans may pay for pill-dispensing technologies that help beneficiaries manage medication, or for a railing to be installed in a bath, which could reduce the risk of hip fractures and complications.[21]

Medicare Advantage Delivers Better Medical Outcomes

Relative to those who remained in traditional Medicare and after controlling for differences in medical risks, seniors who opted for Medicare Advantage managed care plans between 1993 and 1996 were 60 percent less likely to be hospitalized, experienced hospital stays that were 44 percent shorter, and were 14 percent more likely to see a physician at least once during the year.[22]

These numbers do not just reflect differences in the health risks of those enrolled in Medicare Advantage. Even after controlling for observable disparities in medical status, demographics, and geographic location, Medicare Advantage enrollees from 2003 to 2009 experienced 20 percent to 25 percent fewer inpatient hospitalizations and made 25 percent to 35 percent fewer emergency care visits. They also tended to receive more appropriate and cost-effective care. Beneficiaries enrolled in Medicare Advantage managed care plans were more likely to be treated by primary care physicians than by specialists, while heart patients were more likely to receive bypass surgery than percutaneous coronary intervention, reducing the risk that they would require a repeat procedure.[23] Overall, Medicare Advantage patients from 2006 to 2008 were 13 percent to 20 percent less likely to be readmitted to hospital than traditional Medicare enrollees with equivalent diagnoses.[24] The mortality rate of Medicare Advantage enrollees was 33 percent lower than for those in traditional Medicare, with differences in clinical risk factors accounting for a disparity of only 14 percent from 2010 to 2012.[25]

There is evidence to suggest that the adjustment of payments to MA plans for medical diagnoses means that the risks of MA enrollees are better documented than those of other Medicare beneficiaries.[26] To identify the extent of improved health that directly results from increased enrollment in Medicare Advantage, a regression discontinuity study using data from 2009 examined a bump in payments to MA plans in urban areas. Those areas saw an increase in Medicare Advantage enrollment but reduced hospital use and lower rates of mortality.[27]

Medicare Advantage plans also did a better job of providing appropriate care and improving the quality of life for the terminally ill, avoiding overmedicalization with costly, painful, and ineffective procedures at the end of life. In the six months before their deaths, Medicare beneficiaries enrolled in Medicare Advantage between 2003 to 2009 had similar levels of outpatient visits to those in traditional Medicare but were 13 percent to 31 percent more likely to use hospice, 11 percent to 13 percent less likely to be admitted to hospital, and 42 percent to 54 percent less likely to visit the emergency room.[28] Medicare Advantage enrollees were 43 percent less likely than beneficiaries enrolled in traditional Medicare between 2008 and 2010 to die in hospital rather than at home.[29]

In this context, it should be noted that recent research on the comparative performance of Medicare Advantage and traditional Medicare shows that the superior outcomes are not the product of younger and healthier beneficiaries choosing to enroll in Medicare Advantage plans. In fact, the evidence points in the opposite direction. In 2018, Avalere Health reported that MA plans enrolled beneficiaries with greater health risks and a greater likelihood to incur higher costs than beneficiaries enrolled in traditional Medicare. This included a greater number of patients with chronic illnesses and disabilities as well as serious mental illnesses and alcohol and substance abuse.[30]

Medicare Advantage Reduces Medical Costs

The medical costs incurred by beneficiaries enrolled in Medicare Advantage are 25 percent lower than those in the same county and with the same medical risk score as those who are enrolled in traditional Medicare. Even after using differences in mortality to control for unobserved differences in health status (which would underestimate the savings generated by Medicare Advantage to the extent that it reduces mortality), treatment costs for those enrolled in Medicare Advantage are 10 percent lower than under traditional Medicare.[31]

The combination of efficiency gains in procurement and savings from improvements to beneficiaries' health exceed the profits and administrative costs that are incurred by Medicare Advantage plans. For 2020, the cost at which Medicare Advantage plans bid to deliver the standard Medicare package of benefits averaged 12 percent less than traditional Medicare would otherwise have spent.[32]

Medicare Advantage Delivers Better Benefits at Lower Costs

Medicare Advantage plans are allowed to use most of these savings to finance supplemental benefits to attract enrollees, and the enrollee does not pay extra to receive these benefits. Eighty-four percent of Medicare Advantage enrollees received dental benefits—almost always covering preventive exams, x-rays, and cleanings without out-of-pocket costs. Ninety-eight percent of beneficiaries in Medicare Advantage receive additional coverage for free eye exams, while 89 percent get coverage for hearing aids. Many plans also provide access to 24-hour nursing hotlines, telemonitoring, and nonemergency transportation.[33]

Prescription drug coverage is the most popular supplemental benefit for Medicare Advantage to provide. Indeed, private Medicare plans typically covered prescription drugs before Medicare's dedicated Part D prescription drug benefit was even established. Since the enactment of the Part D program, beneficiaries have had the choice of enrolling in stand-alone Part D drug plans or enrolling in Medicare Advantage plans that offer the Part D standardized prescription drug coverage. Enrollment in MA drug plans has outstripped enrollment in stand-alone drug plans. In 2010, for example, 36.3 percent of enrollees were in the MA drug plans. That number jumped to 44.3 percent in 2019, and is projected to be over 50 percent by 2029.[34] Expanded drug coverage attracts enrollees because it reduces the cost of the most prominent routine medical expenses, but it is also because improving access to medications helps to improve the management of chronic conditions and reduce the risk of costly hospitalizations.

The Medicare Part D prescription drug benefit cost beneficiaries enrolled in traditional Medicare an average premium of $505 in 2017, while those enrolled in Medicare Advantage paid an average premium of only $264 that year, and 39 percent of MA enrollees received Part D coverage that required no additional premium at all.[35] Whereas 84 percent of Medicare beneficiaries live in counties where Medicare Advantage plans covering Part D are available for a $0 premium, the lowest available Part D premium for enrollees in traditional Medicare was $175.[36] Medicare Advantage enrollees are therefore significantly more likely to receive prescription drug coverage. Of the beneficiaries not getting Low Income Subsidies or Retiree Drug Subsidies, 50 percent in traditional Medicare and 80 percent in Medicare Advantage were covered by Part D.[37]

The drug coverage that Medicare beneficiaries receive through Medicare Advantage is also significantly more generous. Ninety-eight percent of Medicare Advantage enrollees received drug coverage requiring lower cost sharing than the standard benefit. In contrast, only 42 percent of traditional Medicare enrollees were in Part D drug plans that offered more than basic coverage.[38]

Medicare Advantage plans tend to incorporate clinical nuance to eliminate cost sharing for medications that are most important to managing chronic conditions.[39] Researchers estimate that such approaches reduced enrollees' out-of-pocket drug costs and increased their utilization of drugs relative to those receiving drug coverage through traditional Medicare—with each additional $1 in increased spending on prescription drugs serving to offset other medical costs by $0.20.[40]

Medicare Advantage Delivers Protection from Catastrophic Costs

Medicare Advantage also benefits enrollees by providing them a cap on their out-of-pocket costs and thus solid protection against the financial devastation of catastrophic illness. Medicare Advantage plans are required to limit enrollees' out-of-pocket costs to no more than $6,700 per year, and on average cap them at $5,219.[41] By contrast, traditional Medicare provides no cap on out-of-pocket costs and its cost-sharing structure is a relic of health insurance arrangements from the 1960s. Beneficiaries face a $1,484 deductible for every hospitalization and a separate $201 deductible for physician services. They are also required to pay 20 percent of the cost of Medicare Part B services without limit, which exposes them to tens of thousands of dollars in out-of-pocket costs, often associated with cancer drugs that routinely cost over $100,000 for a course of treatment.[42]

Many traditional Medicare enrollees receive supplemental coverage from previous employers or Medicaid to protect them from catastrophic out-of-pocket costs. Those who do not must purchase supplemental insurance, known as Medigap, whose premiums average $1,824 per year and may not be available to enrollees with preexisting conditions.[43] As poorer Medicare beneficiaries receive cost-sharing assistance through Medicaid and wealthier beneficiaries are able to afford Medigap, Medicare Advantage plans have proven disproportionately popular with middle-income seniors.[44]

Looking Ahead

Since Medicare Advantage was created with the enactment of the Medicare Modernization Act of 2003, Washington policymakers and policy analysts alike have had ample opportunity to witness the success of a defined contribution system of coverage and care. Competitive private health plans, governed by flexible regulation and free to innovate in payment and care delivery, have proven that they can secure better care at lower costs than the highly centralized, bureaucratically controlled, and outdated Medicare fee-for-service program.

• •

CHRISTOPHER POPE, PhD, is a Senior Fellow at the Manhattan Institute.

NOTES

1. Anika L. Hines, Marguerite L. Barrett, H. Joanna Jiang, and Claudia A. Steiner, *Conditions with the Largest Number of Adult Hospital Readmissions by Payer, 2011*, HCUP Statistical Brief no. 172 (Rockville, MD: Agency for Healthcare Research and Quality, April 2014), https://www.hcup-us.ahrq.gov/reports/statbriefs/sb172 -Conditions-Readmissions-Payer.pdf; "National Health Expenditure Data: Historical," Centers for Medicare and Medicaid Services (CMS), accessed December 2020, https://www.cms.gov/Research-Statistics-Data-and-Systems/Statistics-Trends-and -Reports/NationalHealthExpendData/NationalHealthAccountsHistorical.

2. Chris Pope, *Can US Health Care Escape MACRA's Bureaucratic Briar Patch?* (New York: Manhattan Institute, March 28, 2018), https://www.manhattan-institute.org /html/can-us-health-care-escape-macras-bureaucratic-briar-patch-11138.html.

3. MedPAC, *Medicare Advantage Program Payment System* (Washington, DC: Medicare Payment Advisory Committee, November 2021), https://www.medpac .gov/wp-content/uploads/2021/11/medpac_payment_basics_21_ma_final_sec .pdf.

4. According to analysts with Avalere, patients in MA plans had a 29 percent lower rate of potentially avoidable hospitalizations than traditional Medicare. See Dan Mendelson, Christine Teigland, and Sean Creighton, *Medicare Advantage Achieves Cost Effective Care and Better Outcomes for Beneficiaries with Chronic Conditions Relative to Fee-for-Service Medicare* (Washington, DC: Avalere Health, July 2018), 3–4, https://bettermedicarealliance.org/wp-content/uploads/2020/03 /BMA_Avalere_MA_vs_FFS_Medicare_Report_0.pdf.

5. Chris Pope, "Medicare's Single-Payer Experience," *National Affairs* 26 (Winter 2016), https://www.nationalaffairs.com/publications/detail/medicares-single -payer-experience.

6. Michelle M. Stein, "Verma: CMS Has a Long Way to Go to Improve Medicare Program Integrity," *Inside Health Policy*, July 27, 2018, https://insidehealthpolicy.com /daily-news/verma-cms-has-long-way-go-improve-medicare-program-integrity.

7. "2020 Estimated Improper Payment Rates for Centers for Medicare & Medicaid Services (CMS) Programs," *CMS Newsroom*, November 16, 2020, https:// www.cms.gov/newsroom/fact-sheets/2020-estimated-improper-payment-rates -centers-medicare-medicaid-services-cms-programs.

8. Chapin White and Christopher M. Whaley, *Prices Paid to Hospitals by Private Health Plans Are High Relative to Medicare and Vary Widely: Findings from an Employer-Led Transparency Initiative* (Santa Monica, CA: RAND Corporation, 2019), https://www.rand.org/pubs/research_reports/RR3033.html.

9. Erin Trish, Paul Ginsburg, Laura Gascue, and Geoffrey Joyce, "Physician Reimbursement in Medicare Advantage Compared with Traditional Medicare and Commercial Health Insurance," *Journal of the American Medical Association Internal Medicine* 177, no. 9 (September 2017): 1287–95, https://jamanetwork.com/journals /jamainternalmedicine/article-abstract/2643349.

10. Robert A. Berenson, Jonathan H. Sunshine, David Helms, and Emily Lawton, "Why Medicare Advantage Plans Pay Hospitals Traditional Medicare

Prices," *Health Affairs* 34, no. 8 (2015): 1289–95, https://www.healthaffairs.org/doi/full/10.1377/hlthaff.2014.1427.

11. Laurence C. Baker, M. Kate Bundorf, Aileen M. Devlin, and Daniel P. Kessler, "Medicare Advantage Plans Pay Hospitals Less Than Traditional Medicare Pays," *Health Affairs* 35, no. 8 (2016): 1444–51, https://www.healthaffairs.org/doi/full/10.1377/hlthaff.2015.1553.

12. Vilsa Curto, Liran Einav, Amy Finkelstein, Jonathan D. Levin, and Jay Bhattacharya "Healthcare Spending and Utilization in Public and Private Medicare," NBER Working Paper No. 23090 (Cambridge, MA: National Bureau of Economic Research, January 2017), https://www.nber.org/papers/w23090.

13. Joseph P. Newhouse and Thomas G. McGuire, "How Successful Is Medicare Advantage?," *Milbank Quarterly* 92, no. 2 (2014): 351–94, https://www.ncbi.nlm.nih.gov/pmc/articles/PMC4089375/.

14. Newhouse and McGuire, "How Successful Is Medicare Advantage?"

15. John Z. Ayanian, Bruce E. Landon, Alan M. Zaslavsky, Robert C. Saunders, L. Gregory Pawlson, and Joseph P. Newhouse, "Medicare Beneficiaries More Likely to Receive Appropriate Ambulatory Services in HMOs than in Traditional Medicare," *Health Affairs* 32, no. 7 (2013): 1228–35, https://www.healthaffairs.org/doi/full/10.1377/hlthaff.2012.0773.

16. Richard G. Roetzheim, Thomas N. Chirikos, Kristen J. Wells, Ellen P. McCarthy, Long H. Ngo, Donglin Li, Reed E. Drews, and Lisa I. Iezzoni, "Managed Care and Cancer Outcomes for Medicare Beneficiaries with Disabilities," *American Journal of Managed Care* 14, no. 5 (2008): 287–96, https://www.ncbi.nlm.nih.gov/pmc/articles/PMC4110639/.

17. Bruce E. Landon, Alan M. Zaslavsky, Shulamit L. Bernard, Matthew J. Cioffi, and Paul D. Cleary, "Comparison of Performance of Traditional Medicare vs Medicare Managed Care," *Journal of the American Medical Association* 291, no. 14 (2004): 1744–52, https://jamanetwork.com/journals/jama/fullarticle/198537.

18. Emma Goldberg, "UnitedHealth Ships Flu Kits to Medicare Recipients," *New York Times*, October 24, 2020, https://www.nytimes.com/2020/10/24/health/Covid-flu-elderly-Medicare.html.

19. "Humana and Landmark Announce In-Home Care Program for Humana Medicare Advantage Members with Chronic Conditions," Landmark Health, August 24, 2018, https://www.landmarkhealth.org/humana-at-home-care-program/.

20. Robb Cohen, Jeff Lemieux, Jeff Schoenborn, and Teresa Mulligan, "Medicare Advantage Chronic Special Needs Plan Boosted Primary Care, Reduced Hospital Use among Diabetes Patients," *Health Affairs* 31, no. 1 (2012): 110–19, https://www.healthaffairs.org/doi/10.1377/hlthaff.2011.0998.

21. Robert Pear, "Medicare Allows More Benefits for Chronically Ill, Aiming to Improve Care for Millions," *New York Times*, June 24, 2018, https://www.nytimes.com/2018/06/24/us/politics/medicare-chronic-illness-benefits.html.

22. Michelle M. Mello, Sally C. Stearns, and Edward C. Norton, "Do Medicare HMOs Still Reduce Health Services Use after Controlling for Selection Bias?," *Health Economics* 11, no. 5 (2002): 323–40, https://onlinelibrary.wiley.com/doi/abs/10.1002/hec.664.

23. Bruce E. Landon, Alan M. Zaslavsky, Robert C. Saunders, L. Gregory Pawlson, Joseph P. Newhouse, and John Z. Ayanian, "Analysis of Medicare Advantage HMOs Compared with Traditional Medicare Shows Lower Use of Many Services during 2003–09," *Health Affairs* 31, no. 12 (2012): 2609–17, https://www.healthaffairs.org/doi/abs/10.1377/hlthaff.2012.0179.

24. Jeff Lemieux, Cary Sennett, Ray Wang, Teresa Mulligan, and Jon Bumbaugh, "Hospital Readmission Rates in Medicare Advantage Plans," *American Journal of Managed Care* 18, no. 2 (2012): 96–104, https://www.ajmc.com/view/hospital-readmission-rates-in-medicare-advantage-plans.

25. Roy A. Beveridge, Sean M. Mendes, Arial Caplan, Teresa L. Rogstad, Vanessa Olson, Meredith C. Williams, Jacquelyn M. McRae, and Stefan Vargas, "Mortality Differences between Traditional Medicare and Medicare Advantage: A Risk-Adjusted Assessment Using Claims Data," *Inquiry: The Journal of Health Care Organization, Provision, and Financing* 54 (June 2017): 1–8, https://journals.sagepub.com/doi/pdf/10.1177/0046958017709103.

26. Richard Kronick and W. Pete Welch, "Measuring Coding Intensity in the Medicare Advantage Program," *Medicare & Medicaid Research Review* 4, no. 2 (July 17, 2014), https://www.ncbi.nlm.nih.gov/pmc/articles/PMC4109819.

27. Christopher C. Afendulis, Michael E. Chernew, and Daniel P. Kessler, "The Effect of Medicare Advantage on Hospital Admissions and Mortality," *American Journal of Health Economics* 3, no. 2 (2017): 254–79, https://www.journals.uchicago.edu/doi/10.1162/AJHE_a_00074.

28. David G. Stevenson, John Z. Ayanian, Alan M. Zaslavsky, Joseph P. Newhouse, and Bruce E. Landon, "Service Use at the End of Life in Medicare Advantage versus Traditional Medicare," *Medical Care* 51, no. 10 (October 2013): 931–37, https://www.ncbi.nlm.nih.gov/pmc/articles/PMC3804008/.

29. Elizabeth Edmiston Chen and Edward Alan Miller, "A Longitudinal Analysis of Site of Death: The Effects of Continuous Enrollment in Medicare Advantage versus Conventional Medicare," *Research on Aging* 39, no. 8 (2017): 960–86, https://journals.sagepub.com/doi/abs/10.1177/0164027516645843.

30. Mendelson, Teigland, and Creighton, *Medicare Advantage Achieves Cost Effective Care and Better Outcomes*, 4.

31. Vilsa Curto et al., "Healthcare Spending and Utilization in Public and Private Medicare."

32. MedPAC, "The Medicare Advantage Program: Status Report," chapter 13 in *Report to the Congress: Medicare Payment Policy* (Washington, DC: Medicare Payment Advisory Commission, March 2020), 376, table 13.3, https://www.medpac.gov/wp-content/uploads/import_data/scrape_files/docs/default-source/reports/mar20_medpac_ch13_sec.pdf. Hereafter cited as "Medicare Advantage Status Report."

33. Christopher Pope, "Supplemental Benefits under Medicare Advantage," *Health Affairs Blog*, January 21, 2016, https://www.healthaffairs.org/do/10.1377 /hblog20160121.052787/full/; Julia M. Friedman and Mary G. Yeh, "Prevalence of Supplemental Benefits in the General Enrollment Medicare Advantage Market- place: 2017 to 2021" (white paper, Milliman, December 2020), https://www .milliman.com/-/media/milliman/pdfs/2020-articles/articles/12-14-20 -prevalence_of_supplemental_benefits_general_enrollment-v1.ashx.

34. Boards of Trustees of the Federal Hospital Insurance and the Supple- mentary Medical Insurance Trust Funds, *2020 Annual Report of the Boards of Trustees* (Washington, DC: Centers for Medicare and Medicaid Services, April 22, 2020), 139–40, https://www.cms.gov/files/document/2020-medicare -trustees-report.pdf.

35. CMS, "Medicare Current Beneficiary Survey," December 2020, https://www .cms.gov/Research-Statistics-Data-and-Systems/Research/MCBS; CMS, "Medicare Current Beneficiary Survey," 2017.

36. MedPAC, "Medicare Advantage Status Report"; CMS, "Medicare Current Beneficiary Survey," March 2018.

37. CMS, "Medicare Current Beneficiary Survey," 2017. See also Chris Pope, *Protecting Seniors from High Drug Costs* (New York: Manhattan Institute, March 23, 2021), https://www.manhattan-institute.org/protecting-seniors-high-drug-costs.

38. MedPAC, "The Medicare Prescription Drug Program (Part D): Status Report," chapter 14 in *Report to the Congress: Medicare Payment Policy* (Washington, DC: Medicare Payment Advisory Commission, March 2020), 418, https://www .medpac.gov/wp-content/uploads/import_data/scrape_files/docs/default-source /reports/mar20_medpac_ch14_sec.pdf.

39. Michael E. Chernew and A. Mark Fendrick, "Improving Benefit Design to Promote Effective, Efficient, and Affordable Care," *Journal of the American Medical Association* 316, no. 16 (2016): 1651–52, https://jamanetwork.com/journals/jama /article-abstract/2556007; "The Role of Value-Based Insurance Design in Medicare Advantage Plans," Center for Value-Based Insurance Design, accessed Decem- ber 2020, https://vbidcenter.org/initiatives/medicare-and-medicare-advantage.

40. Amanda Starc and Robert J. Town, "Internalizing Behavioral Externalities: Benefit Integration in Health Insurance," NBER Working Paper No. 21783 (Cambridge, MA: National Bureau of Economic Research, December 2015), https://www.nber.org/system/files/working_papers/w21783/revisions/w21783 .rev0.pdf.

41. "Medicare Fact Sheet: Medicare Advantage," Kaiser Family Foundation, June 6, 2019, https://www.kff.org/medicare/fact-sheet/medicare-advantage/.

42. Hagop Kantarjian, David Steensma, Judit Rius Sanjuan, Adam Elshaug, and Donald Light, "High Cancer Drug Prices in the United States: Reasons and Proposed Solutions," *Journal of Oncology Practice* 10, no. 4 (2014): e208–11, https://ascopubs.org/doi/full/10.1200/jop.2013.001351.

43. "How Much Does a Medicare Supplement Insurance Plan Cost?," eHealth, October 24, 2018, https://www.ehealthinsurance.com/medicare/supplement-all/how

-much-medicare-supplement-plans-cost; Cristina Boccuti, Gretchen Jacobson, Kendal Orgera, and Tricia Neuman, "Medigap Enrollment and Consumer Protections Vary across States," Kaiser Family Foundation, July 11, 2018, https://www.kff.org/medicare /issue-brief/medigap-enrollment-and-consumer-protections-vary-across-states/.

44. Chris Pope, *Enhancing Medicare Advantage* (New York: Manhattan Institute, February 28, 2019), https://www.manhattan-institute.org/medicare-advantage -better-than-traditional-medicare.

Improving Medicare Advantage through Patient Power

The Medicare Advantage (MA) program has been immensely successful in attracting large numbers of buyers and sellers into what has become a vibrant, competitive market for senior health care. We have barely scratched the surface, however, in liberating market forces.[1] Although the Trump administration did much to reform the entire Medicare program,[2] too many regulations and bureaucratic barriers still impede normal market processes. The program can be made better in the aspects of improving health care for the beneficiaries; removing provider obstacles to timely, high-quality care; and saving money for patients and taxpayers.[3]

Giving Patients the Power to Manage Their Own Health Care Budgets

Almost all Medicare dollars go to someone other than the patient. As a result, the medical marketplace for the elderly and the disabled tends to be more bureaucratic and less responsive to customer preferences than markets where customers buy goods and services with their own money. By contrast, federal tax policy allows young people to have a health savings account (HSA) that they own and manage. Deposits to these accounts are before-tax, and if the funds are spent on health care, they are never taxed. The advantage of such a system is that self-insurance (by means of the savings account) is, under the tax law, on a level playing field with third-party health insurance purchased through an employer. Decisions about which medical services will be purchased by the patient and which will be purchased by a third party are made based on individual preferences[4] and supply-side opportunities, not on distortions created by the income tax system.[5] Once seniors become eligible for Medicare, however, they are no longer able to make deposits to HSAs. Nor can they have a similarly functioning health reimbursement arrangement (HRA),[6] unless it is created by an employer.[7]

Part of the reason for this disparate treatment is the complexities of tax law. Health insurance and savings accounts for young people are intricately tied up with the tax law in arcane ways. Health insurance for seniors, by contrast, is either untaxed or after-tax. Medicare benefits, for example, are not taxed at all. And senior premiums for Medicare Parts B, C, and D and for Medigap insurance are all paid with after-tax money.

Accounts that seniors own and control need to be integrated with the rest of Medicare. Accounts that potentially do this best are called Roth HSAs. If Congress allowed a Medicare Advantage plan to make a deposit to such an account, the funds would not be taxed at the time of deposit or when they are withdrawn for any purpose. Also, when seniors make their own deposits to these accounts, the deposits would be made with after-tax dollars and the withdrawals (for any purpose) would be tax-free.[8]

Roth HSAs, therefore, are a way of using the tax law to encourage health insurance for the elderly and the disabled without distorting any important decisions. The choice between self-insurance and third-party insurance would be made on a level playing field under the tax law. The choice between spending out of the account on health care or on nonhealth goods and services would also be made on a level playing field. And the choice between spending from the account on anything in the current period and spending on health and nonhealth in all future periods would also be unimpeded by tax law distortions.

Empowering Chronically Ill Patients

Although they serve many useful purposes, HSAs in operation today are governed by far too many restrictions. In general, one cannot have an account unless it is combined with third-party insurance with an across-the-board deductible. Under the most common arrangement, HSA funds are available to pay some or all medical expenses below the deductible, and third-party health insurance pays for everything above it. Money not spent from the account grows tax-free.

This is an ideal account for healthy people, who have only occasional expenses for minor medical problems. For these people, the account functions mainly as a savings account. However, for a chronically ill patient with, say, $3,000 or $4,000 of routine expenses every year, the account is of very limited value.

It is estimated that chronic illness is responsible for as much as 75 percent of all health care spending.[9] Yet almost nowhere in the entire health care system is there a mechanism for chronically ill patients to manage their own health care dollars.

One highly successful exception to this observation is the Medicaid Cash and Counseling Program.[10] Started several decades ago, this program originally allowed those who are homebound and disabled the right to manage their own budgets. That meant they had the right to hire and fire the people who serviced them, and any money saved could be spent in other ways that benefited themselves. Satisfaction rates in this program were in the mid-90s percentile (something rarely seen in any health program anywhere in the world).[11] And because of this success, the program has been expanded. Today, for example, the family of an Alzheimer's patient can receive a budget to manage the patient's care.

We need to expand this idea to all forms of chronic care. Studies show that chronic patients can often manage their own care as well or better than traditional doctor care, with minimal patient education.[12] If they are to be allowed to manage their own care, they should be allowed to manage the dollars that pay for that care.[13]

No patient should be forced to do this. But in return for a patient's willingness to manage their own care, Medicare Advantage plans should be able to put money into an account controlled by the patient themself.

Like the current plans paired with HSAs, Medicare Advantage plans should be able to create a high-deductible arrangement under which enrollees manage and pay for expenses below the deductible, and the plan pays for everything above it. Unlike the overly regulated and overly complicated HSA plans for young people, MA organizations should be able to make their own decisions about which expenses are subject to the deductible and which are not.

We shouldn't limit the idea to chronic care, however. As the following examples show, Medicare Advantage plans should be able to carve out entire areas of care and put funds into accounts that patients can manage to pay for that care.[14]

Harnessing the Power of Virtual Medicine

The benefits of telemedicine have been long known.[15] But as we entered the year 2020, it was generally illegal (by act of Congress) for doctors to charge Medicare for a patient consultation by means of phone, email, or Skype.

Two things made radical change possible: the onset of COVID-19 and the Trump administration's response to it.[16] Legalizing telemedical care was not a simple act. There are roughly 7,500 procedures Medicare pays doctors to do. The Centers for Medicare and Medicaid Services (CMS) had to sort through those and determine which were candidates for virtual medicine and which were not. Fortunately, CMS had been sorting through those problems in the first three years of the Trump administration—including pushing the limits of the congressional restrictions and allowing great leeway in the Medicare Advantage program.[17] So when COVID struck, the administration was ready to unleash telehealth in a major way. Congress was only too willing to let the administration do what it wanted to do all along.

The change in the behavior of doctors and patients has been nothing short of breathtaking. According to CMS, between March and June of 2020, more than 9 million Medicare beneficiaries received a telehealth service (including 22 percent of beneficiaries who live in rural areas and almost one in three beneficiaries who live in cities).[18] All the more remarkable as seniors are the least computer-literate segment of the population.

Unfortunately, none of these changes are permanent. The administration's executive orders can easily be reversed by a future president. And new congressional authority is in almost every case tied to the COVID threat. When the virus goes away, the newly acquired freedoms we just described are scheduled to also go away. Congress needs to codify these changes and ensure their permanence.

Creating Access to 24-7 Primary Care

The ability to talk with a doctor by phone or email or Skype—day or night and on weekends—used to be a privilege only the rich could afford. We used to call it "concierge care." The benefits are obvious. The coronavirus and other medical problems don't just crop up during working hours. And a trip to the emergency room is not only expensive but waiting in a room full of other sick people has health risks as well.

Today, Atlas MD, a practice in Wichita, Kansas, reports that it can provide seniors with all primary care, including in-person and round-the-clock care, by means of phone, email, Skype, Zoom, and Facebook, if needed—for $100 a month.[19] That's less than seniors are paying for their Medicare Part B premium. So, it's possible that Medicare Advantage plans could make this kind of arrangement available for a small monthly fee or perhaps no fee at all.

This type of care is generally called "direct primary care" (DPC), and it needs to be an option in regular Medicare as well as in the MA program. Direct primary care doctors not only offer patients the entire range of primary care services, but they also help patients make appointments with specialists, help get discount prices on MRI scans and other medical tests, and provide generic drugs for less than Medicaid pays, in some instances.

One option currently open to Medicare Advantage plans is to offer direct primary care as part of the package of benefits available to their enrollees. However, it appears that most DPC doctors do not want to have a relationship with third-party payers (especially Medicare); in many cases that is why they are DPC doctors in the first place. If Medicare patients had a Roth HSA, however, they could overcome that hurdle by making their own arrangements with non-Medicare doctors.

Patient control of primary care dollars would also open up other opportunities. For example, a Medicare Advantage plan might make a monthly deposit to a Roth account for a patient who prefers to self-manage all of her primary care. Instead of calling a DPC doctor, the patient might call a telehealth physician instead.[20] Or rather than a telemedical consultation with a DPC doctor on nights and weekends, the patient might take advantage of an Uber-type house call service.[21] In other words, some patients might decide they can get better care and cheaper care by taking advantage of the different primary care services that are emerging in the marketplace.

Rewarding Patients for Making Cost-Saving Choices

One of the ways employers are holding down costs and encouraging employees to be price-conscious in the medical marketplace is by a technique called "reference pricing."[22] The employer, for example, might set a price for a medical test, or even a certain kind of surgery, and limit the employer's exposure to that price. Employees are free to choose providers who charge more, but the extra fee must be paid out of the employee's pocket.

In one very notable example, California state employees, retirees, and their families were told that the limit on hip and knee surgery would be $30,000.[23] They were also given a list of 40 or so hospitals that met quality standards and routinely performed the surgery for that fee or less. Employees were free to contract with any provider and initially about one-third went "out of network" and paid higher fees when they did so. Within two years, however, the average out-of-network charge fell to below $30,000.

What makes this example so striking is that we are often told that the only way to get costs down is through the buying power of a large purchaser. In this case, the large buyer (the state) sat idly by while individual buyers, concerned about their own finances, got better deals than large insurers, and even the state of California, were getting elsewhere.

Unfortunately, the way reference pricing is practiced these days, all the incentives are negative. Employees who pay above the reference price are penalized with extra costs, but there is no reward for employees who choose providers who charge less than the reference prices and save money for everyone.

That needs to change across the board, starting in Medicare. Congress, for example, could allow Roth HSAs to be a repository for savings that patients help generate. Such an approach would allow all Medicare enrollees, not just members of Medicare Advantage plans, to have an account they can add to whenever they save money for Medicare.

This principle is especially important if we want patients to take advantage of the opportunities created by medical tourism.[24] We know that Canadian patients who come to the United States for hip and knee replacements get package prices that are about half of what private insurers pay. There is nothing that Canadian patients do that American patients cannot also do, however, provided they are willing to travel.

Under the current system the only entities that can take advantage of the savings created by medical tourism without paying tax penalties are employers, insurance companies, and the government.[25] We need to add Medicare patients to that list.

Rewarding Patients for Healthy Behavior

The single biggest factor in the successful treatment of chronic illness is usually patient compliance. Patients who adhere to their prescription drug routine and who follow their doctor's advice in other ways tend to get better. Those who do not comply tend to get worse. Noncompliance is not only bad for the patient's health, but it also raises costs for the health plan. That means it raises cost for all the other enrollees.

One way a Medicare Advantage plan might handle this problem is with financial incentives. Patients who manage their own health care dollars in a Roth account, for example, would directly pay the cost of noncompliance and reap financial benefits when they do comply. Plans should be able to create similar economic incentives for enrollees who are not managing their own accounts.

Creating a Market for Patient Care

In a normal market, low-cost producers tend to win out in competition with high-cost producers. For the same price, better quality products outsell lower quality. Unfortunately, these normal market forces have been suppressed in the Medicare Advantage program. Patients would be better off if health plans could engage in mutually beneficial exchanges with each other and with the patients themselves.

Suppose that Plan A has the same outcomes for heart patients as Plan B, but Plan A achieves these results at a lower cost. Then there is a social gain to be had if patients could conveniently move from B to A. How could that be done?

Suppose that Medicare's risk-adjusted payment is so low that both plans are losing money on heart patients.[26] Since B's losses are greater than A's, both plans can gain (the combined loss will be less) if B pays A to take all of B's heart patients.

Suppose that Medicare's risk-adjusted payment is high enough to allow both plans to profit from heart care. Since A's profits are greater, both plans can gain (the combined profit will be greater) if A pays B to take all of B's heart patients.

Patients wouldn't have to change plans if they prefer not to. So, to induce them to make changes, plans should be able to offer something to the patients—say, a premium reduction, a deposit to a health savings account, or extra benefits.

Similar reasoning applies where there are quality differences— especially differences that are reflected in higher Medicare payments to plans that achieve higher quality scores. A mutually beneficial transfer of patients from low-quality plans to high-quality plans for a particular disease category has the potential to make all plans and all patients better off.

Allowing the Right Patient into the Right Plan

A market for the chronically ill would work best if there were no restrictions on the ability of patients to enter the plan that best fits their needs. When their medical needs change, a change of plans is often advisable. Unfortunately, in the current system that's not always easy. When beneficiaries can enroll in a Medicare Advantage plan, when they can switch plans, and how often they can switch are subject to a hodgepodge of complicated, confusing restrictions that we won't try to summarize here.

When the Medicare Advantage program was first started, critics feared that patient movement might destabilize the market. Suppose one plan got a reputation for being very good at cancer care. Then, the minute patients were diagnosed with cancer, they might all rush over and join that plan. All the heart patients might converge on another plan. Ditto for diabetes or any other ailment. That fear is no longer a serious worry, though, and the reason is Medicare Advantage has the most sophisticated risk adjustment system in the world. Medicare Advantage is the only place in our health care system where a health plan can send in new information from a patient's medical records and get an adjustment in the premium it receives. In making the premium decision, Medicare uses more than 70 different variables to make sure the plan gets an actuarially fair premium based on a patient's medical condition. That is not to say the risk adjustment program cannot be improved, but MA's stellar progress in this area cannot be overlooked.

Medicare is also the only place in our health care system where health plans can specialize in diseases, such as heart disease, lung disease, diabetes, and so on. And the plans can advertise their specialty. They can ask medical questions at the point of entry and they can request medical records.

Much more could be done. As a rule, health records should always travel with patients wherever they go. And all plans, not just special needs plans, should be able to ask medical questions. Getting the right patient into the right plan should be a goal built into the system, not something that just occasionally happens.

Beyond Medicare Advantage: Empowering Patients in Traditional Medicare

At last count, there were 10.4 million Medicare beneficiaries connected to an accountable care organization (ACO). Although these enrollees have been encouraged to think they are participating in traditional fee-for-service Medicare, they are in fact being treated by physicians who face economic incentives like those of a traditional HMO (health maintenance organization). Unlike Medicare Advantage plans, which generally have lower costs and higher quality ratings than traditional Medicare, the ACO experiment has been largely disappointing. Without the tools routinely used by Medicare Advantage plans, ACOs are neither saving money in the aggregate nor are they improving the quality of care.[27]

Until the Trump administration made changes, ACO doctors were muzzled. They were not allowed to tell their patients they were participating in an ACO. Even today they are not allowed to encourage their patients to join a Medicare Advantage plan with which they are affiliated. And they face criminal penalties if they offer their patients economic incentives to join their Medicare Advantage plan.

These are the wrong rules and the wrong incentives. We should be encouraging patients to move from plans that are higher-cost and lower-quality to plans that do a better job across the board. Since there are social gains to be had from a migration of patients from ACOs to Medicare Advantage plans, Washington policymakers should give their blessing to economic incentives, such as those discussed in this chapter, that encourage that change.

Protecting the Right of Return

Medicare Advantage plan enrollees have the right to leave their Medicare Advantage plan and enroll in traditional Medicare. When they do so they should not be penalized by the current Medigap insurance market rules that discourage that enrollment, particularly if they have maintained continuous Medicare Advantage coverage. Supplemental Medicare insurance (Medigap policies) fills in the gaps of coverage in conventional Medicare. Under current regulations, these plans charge everyone the same premium, regardless of health status, as long as they enroll when they are first eligible. Failure to promptly enroll can result in higher premiums and the longer the wait, the higher the charge. In some states, late comers can be medically underwritten and face premiums that reflect their health status. Medicare Advantage enrollees should be protected from these penalties if they decide to return to conventional Medicare.

Looking Ahead

Medicare Advantage has been a rare health policy success. Its rapid growth in recent years is attributable to its strong integrated benefits package with catastrophic protection, the variety of competitive health plan options, and its ability to provide better care at lower costs. It is the exercise of patient choice that fueled Medicare Advantage's successes, and the power of patients to make even more decisions could lead to further improvements should Congress enable them to use health savings accounts, control their own budgets, and take advantage of modern information technology and the advances in the provision of primary care.

· ·

JOHN C. GOODMAN is president of the Goodman Institute for Public Policy Research and author of *New Way to Care* (Independent Institute, 2020).

NOTES
1. Thomas Saving and John C. Goodman, "A Better Way to Approach Medicare's Impossible Task," *Health Affairs Blog*, November 15, 2011, https://www.healthaffairs.org/do/10.1377/hblog20111115.015114/full.

2. US Department of Health and Human Services, US Department of the Treasury, and US Department of Labor, *Reforming America's Healthcare System through Choice and Competition*, December 2018, https://www.hhs.gov/sites/default/files/Reforming-Americas-Healthcare-System-Through-Choice-and-Competition.pdf.

3. John C. Goodman and Lawrence J. Wedekind, "How the Trump Administration Is Reforming Medicare," *Health Affairs Blog*, May 3, 2019, https://www.healthaffairs.org/do/10.1377/hblog20190501.529581/full/; John C. Goodman and Lawrence J. Wedekind, "How Trump Is Reforming Medicare, Part II," *Forbes*, July 12, 2019, https://www.forbes.com/sites/johngoodman/2019/07/12/how-trump-is-reforming-medicare-part-ii.

4. Individuals, spending their own money, can sometimes obtain lower prices and higher quality than purchases made by third-party payer bureaucracies.

5. Under current law, employer contributions to an employee health plan are made with pretax dollars. However, out-of-pocket spending by the employee is made with after-tax dollars. This gives employees a distorted incentive to "buy" health care through their employer's plan instead of receiving more compensation as taxable wages and buying care on their own. When deposits to an HSA are made with pretax dollars, the two types of spending will be on a level playing field. Decisions about how to purchase care, therefore, will not be biased by the tax code.

6. Under an HRA, employees can draw on an employer-funded account to purchase health care services. Unlike an HSA, however, they cannot withdraw unspent funds for other, non–health care purposes.

7. John C. Goodman, "Saving for Health Care: The Policy Pros and Cons of Different Vehicles," *Health Affairs Blog*, April 17, 2012, https://www.healthaffairs.org/do/10.1377/hblog20120417.017858/full.

8. Mark V. Pauly, John C. Goodman, Judith Feder, Larry Levitt, Stuart M. Butler, David M. Cutler, and Gail R. Wilensky, "Tax Credits for Health Insurance and Medical Savings Accounts," *Health Affairs* 14, no.1 (1995): 125–39, https://www.healthaffairs.org/doi/full/10.1377/hlthaff.14.1.125.

9. Partnership to Fight Chronic Disease, "Fighting Chronic Disease: The Case for Enhancing the Congressional Budget Analysis Process," accessed January 29, 2021, https://www.fightchronicdisease.org/sites/default/files/docs/PFCD_ChronDisease_FactSheet3Final.pdf.

10. "Cash & Counseling Programs: Get Paid as a Family Caregiver," Paying for Senior Care, updated August 21, 2019, https://www.payingforseniorcare.com/paid-caregiver/cash-and-counseling-program.

11. John C. Goodman, "An International Trend toward Self-Directed Care," *Health Affairs Blog*, April 9, 2010, https://www.healthaffairs.org/do/10.1377/hblog20100409.004702/full.

12. Anna Gorman, "With Chronic Illness, You Are Your Own Best Friend," *Kaiser Health News*, September 7, 2016, https://khn.org/news/with-chronic-illness-you-are-your-own-best-friend.

13. John C. Goodman, "Patient Power for Chronic Illness," *Health Affairs Blog*, February 12, 2009, https://www.healthaffairs.org/do/10.1377/hblog20090212.000502/full.

14. John C. Goodman, Gerald L. Musgrave, and Devon M. Herrick, "Designing Ideal Health Insurance," in *Lives at Risk: Single-Payer National Health Insurance around the World* (Lanham, MD: Rowman & Littlefield, 2004), 235–53, http://www.ncpathinktank.org/pdfs/livesatrisk/Ch24.pdf.

15. John C. Goodman, "Lower Cost, Higher Quality Health Care Is Right at Our Fingertips," *Forbes*, July 23, 2018, https://www.forbes.com/sites/johngoodman/2018/07/23/lower-cost-higher-quality-health-care-is-right-at-our-fingertips.

16. John C. Goodman and Marie Fishpaw, "What Trump Has Done to Change Health Care and How It's Helped Battle COVID-19," *National Review*, October 18, 2020, https://www.nationalreview.com/2020/10/what-trump-has-done-to-change-the-health-care-system-and-how-that-has-helped-battle-covid-19.

17. Centers for Medicare and Medicaid Services, "CMS Proposes Historic Changes to Modernize Medicare and Restore the Doctor-Patient Relationship," press release, July 12, 2018, https://www.cms.gov/newsroom/press-releases/cms-proposes-historic-changes-modernize-medicare-and-restore-doctor-patient-relationship.

18. Rajiv Leventhal, "CMS' Verma Touts Telehealth Success during Pandemic; Taskforce to Work on Policy Recommendations," *Healthcare Innovation*, July 23, 2020, https://www.hcinnovationgroup.com/population-health-management/telehealth/news/21147369/cms-verma-touts-telehealth-success-during-pandemic-taskforce-to-work-on-policy-recommendations.

19. "Atlas MD: Our Fees," Atlas MD, accessed January 29, 2021, https://atlas.md/wichita.

20. Goodman, "Lower Cost, Higher Quality Health Care Is Right at Our Fingertips."

21. John C. Goodman, "What Does Uber Medicine Look Like?," *Forbes*, July 24, 2015, https://www.forbes.com/sites/johngoodman/2015/07/24/what-does-uber-medicine-look-like.

22. Ann Boynton and James C. Robinson, "Appropriate Use of Reference Pricing Can Increase Value," *Health Affairs Blog*, July 7, 2015, https://www.healthaffairs.org/do/10.1377/hblog20150707.049155/full.

23. John Goodman, "Stunning Results from California," *Health Policy Blog*, August 7, 2013, http://healthblog.ncpathinktank.org/stunning-results-from-california.

24. Devon M. Herrick, *Medical Tourism: Global Competition in Health Care*, NCPA Policy Report no. 304 (Dallas, TX: National Center for Policy Analysis, November 2007), http://www.ncpathinktank.org/pub/st304.

25. If employers share savings with employees under the current system, those payments will be treated as taxable income to the employees.

26. As noted, Medicare pays Medicare Advantage plans a premium for each enrollee that is based on the enrollee's health status.

27. Goodman and Wedekind, "How the Trump Administration Is Reforming Medicare."

• CHAPTER 6   Brian J. Miller, MD, and Gail R. Wilensky, PhD

The Next Step in Medicare Reform

Accounting for one-fifth of national health spending, Medicare plays a major role in structuring our nation's health system.[1] Like other fee-for-service (FFS) health plans over the past half-century, Medicare has failed at both cost control and integrating or coordinating benefits for retirement-age Americans. With retirees (many with multimorbidity) set to outnumber children under 18 by 2035,[2] a high importance should be placed on rethinking health care financing and delivery. The payment system behind traditional Medicare (Parts A and B) directly reimburses clinicians on the basis of the number of services delivered and is at the center of the debate on how policymakers can incentivize efficient, high-value care to beneficiaries.

Under a pay-for-volume system, an unlimited number of services could be delivered with no cost ceiling, presenting Medicare as a blank check for the health care of nearly 67 million Americans.[3] Democrats[4] and Republicans[5] alike have questioned the sustainability of federal spending on health care programs, which is projected to steadily rise as a percentage of gross domestic product over the next 30 years.[6]

This chapter reviews the history of insurance design in the Medicare program, including the challenges of insurance design and subsequent application of risk transfer tools in traditional FFS Medicare. Alongside this evolution, we characterize the introduction and growth of private plans in the Medicare marketplace, noting benefits and trade-offs for both beneficiaries and taxpayers. Finally, utilizing lessons from retirement planning, we recommend Congress auto-enroll newly eligible beneficiaries into Medicare Advantage (MA), with a default assignment into the lowest cost (i.e., zero premium) plan. Such a change would provide policymakers with a potential framework to help stabilize program budgeting by placing more beneficiaries into risk-adjusted, capitated plan products.

Insurance Design in the Medicare Program

The Medicare program consists of two primary programs: traditional Medicare (a FFS model) and Medicare Advantage, which is based on market-driven health plan competition. The FFS model, consisting of two-thirds of the Medicare market, is a product of insurance design dating back to its legislative birth in the 1960s, while MA emerged in the 1970s and has tracked the rise of the managed care industry. Here we briefly review the design of, periodic updates to, and challenges of each.

Traditional Medicare and the Evolution
of a Publicly Funded FFS System

Originating in the Social Security Amendments Act of 1965 (H.R. 6675), Medicare began its life as a traditional FFS health plan with the aim of providing coverage to impoverished elderly Americans in the remaining few years of their life; average life expectancy at birth was 70.5 years.[7] Like other FFS plans, Medicare relied on price regulation for cost control. Health economists typically describe the "health care cost equation," in which total cost is a function of price, volume, and the intensity of service,[8] or f (P,V,I) (fig. 6.1). For traditional Medicare, the Centers for Medicare and Medicare Services (CMS)

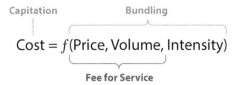

FIGURE 6.1. Health Care Cost Equation. The "health care cost equation" shows cost as a function of price, volume, and intensity of health care. Capitation, which covers the total cost of health care, is similar to bundling in that they both address all three of these elements (capitation addresses the total cost of care, while bundling focuses on an episode of care). By contrast, fee-for-service fails to address intensity of care. *Source*: Brian J. Miller, "Regulation & Principles of Health Insurance," lecture at Kenan-Flagler Business School on April 12, 2019.

administratively sets prices for physician and hospital services, while clinicians and beneficiaries jointly determine the volume and intensity of services.

With administratively set prices,[9] traditional Medicare implicitly rewards clinicians on the basis of volume while intensity of care remains insufficiently addressed, a policy failure characterized by repeated congressional attempts at reform.

Recognizing the challenges of budgetary control within a FFS context,[10] the Reagan administration and Congress worked together to craft legislation to introduce prospective payment and episodic bundling for hospital care. The diagnosis-related group (DRG) system, introduced in 1983 as part of the Social Security amendments,[11] implemented a prospective payment system anchored by hospitalization and including associated costs (service, pharmaceuticals, devices, etc.). A patient's principal diagnosis and up to 24 secondary diagnoses— including comorbidities or complications—determine the DRG category, which determines the base payment rate,[12] an amount further adjusted for geographic variation in wages, graduate medical education, and other features such as rural location.[13]

Following implementation, hospitals could no longer bill based upon incurred costs: prospective, bundled payment initially drove efficiency gains. Over time, hospitals began to shift services to the outpatient setting, in part to escape DRG-based payment. Recognizing this,

Congress—as part of the Omnibus Budget Reconciliation Act of 1990—created a "three-day payment window," mandating inclusion of hospital outpatient services in the DRG payment bundle if provided within the three days prior to hospital admission. While areas such as hospice have retained a per diem (daily) rate,[14] other components of traditional Medicare, such as home health[15] and outpatient hospital services,[16] have transitioned to episodic, prospective payment systems.

For physician payment, the CMS has attempted to deploy other tools of risk transfer in order to drive performance.[17] The Medicare Access and CHIP Reauthorization Act of 2015 (MACRA) created two quality performance pathways for physicians: an alternative payment model (APM) and the merit-based incentive payment system (MIPS), with practices choosing their "path to risk." Practices could opt to receive a 5 percent payment boost for participating in an APM through the CMS Innovation Center. Alternatively, physicians could participate in MIPS, a risk corridor with scoring in multiple areas. Summed and weighted performance across measured areas dictates payment adjustment, a risk corridor of +/− 9 percent for payment year (PY) 2020.[18]

In theory, health plans can choose both the metrics and adjust the "performance bar" annually. The CMS is no exception, although it is statutorily constrained in that MACRA specified that the combination of bonuses and penalties must remain budget neutral. Based upon PY 2018 data, 97 percent of practices received a positive score and a bonus payment, with 84 percent of practices demonstrating "exceptional performance" and achieving the maximum payment adjustment of +1.68 percent,[19] suggesting the metrics driving the risk corridor are inadequately anchored to performance.

The evolution of FFS Medicare reflects the application of multiple tools from policymakers' payment policy tool kit. Risk corridors tie percentage payment adjustments to performance metrics, noting that providers can game metrics or plans can anchor performance targets too low, failing to meaningfully drive performance, as in the case of MIPS. Episodic bundles triggered by clinical events such as inpatient admission or elective surgeries capitate risk across an event or time yet are subject to other forms of gaming. For decades, under DRG-based reimbursements, hospitals have benefited from readmissions, a more recent target of CMS quality efforts.

While the Medicare FFS model of the twenty-first century deploys more tools of risk transfer than Medicare in its original form, it still suffers from uncontrolled cost growth.[20] Unlike private plans, traditional FFS cost control mechanisms, such as prior authorization and utilization review, remain reviled by physicians and unfeasible politically. Network design is absent: Medicare represents an "any-willing provider" network,[21] wherein a beneficiary can see any physician regardless of their quality or cost-effectiveness. Other tools of cost control, such as partial and full capitation, which serve to transfer both financial and clinical risk from payers to providers, remain undeployed (see fig. 6.2.)

The limitations and struggles with cost growth in FFS Medicare served as the impetus for the entrance of and simultaneous development of managed care plans in Medicare.

The Role of Private Plans in the Medicare Program

While their initial involvement in the Medicare market began inauspiciously as cost contracts, through continued legislative attention and

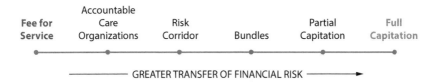

FIGURE 6.2. Spectrum of Risk Transfer. By its nature as a defined contribution, Medicare Advantage exemplifies full capitation and moves the health care system along "the path to value." Other policy interventions, such as ACOs and risk corridors, are less complete. *Source*: Brian J. Miller, "Regulation & Principles of Health Insurance," lecture at Kenan-Flagler Business School on April 12, 2019.

industry innovation, private plans now comprise more than one-third of Medicare's total enrollment. Throughout the 1970s, private markets continued experimenting with health maintenance organization (HMO)–style plans, spurred by both growing costs and the HMO Act of 1973.[22] The Medicare program was no exception, with the Tax Equity and Fiscal Responsibility Act of 1982 creating a pathway for HMOs in Medicare. Plans were capitated and prospectively paid 95 percent of the adjusted average capita cost, with payment adjusted for demographic, disability, institutional, and Medicaid status. Enrollment lagged due to a lack of consumer familiarity with network plans and statutory limitations on plan design.

After slow growth in the 1990s, Congress passed the Balanced Budget Act of 1997, transforming private Medicare by expanding the choice of product offerings and—in an attempt to improve payment accuracy—requiring changes to risk adjustment methodologies. Renamed Medicare+Choice, plans could now offer additional designs, including preferred provider organizations (PPOs), private FFS, medical savings accounts, and provider-sponsored organization plans. This expansion of beneficiary choice was, however, countered by changes in payment methodologies, driving plan exit from many county-level markets.[23]

Congress responded with the 2003 Medicare Modernization Act (MMA), creating the Medicare prescription drug benefit (Part D), authorizing special needs plans (SNPs) for further plan customization, and modifying plan payment methodology. MMA implementation coincided with a wave of retirees who, both comfortable and experienced with network plans offered by their employers, enrolled in MA in droves.[24] As part of implementing the 2010 Affordable Care Act (ACA), the CMS enacted a final adjustment based upon academic research demonstrating overpayment of MA plans,[25] further modifying plan payment methodology to bring MA in line with FFS spending while simultaneously tying the Star Ratings quality program to payment bonuses,[26] resulting in the Medicare Advantage program that exists today.

Beneficiary Trade-offs in Medicare Advantage

Medicare Advantage, as it exists today, represents a series of trade-offs for both beneficiaries and policymakers. Beneficiaries gain limitation on their personal financial liability along with supplemental benefits, both in exchange for some utilization and network controls for health care products and services.

In 2019, the average premium of MA plans (paid for as a separate cost to those of Part A and B) is estimated to be 7.2 percent ($4.50) cheaper than the basic Part D premium alone (which traditional Medicare beneficiaries purchase separately).[27] Further, in 2019, half of MA beneficiaries had a "zero premium" plan,[28] and average premiums are expected to decrease by 23 percent in 2020.[29]

MA plans also set limits on out-of-pocket costs to consumers, unlike its FFS alternative. For HMOs that cover in-network services, this limit averaged $5,059 for 2019 and could not exceed $6,700. PPOs, which offer coverage for both in-network and out-of-network providers, must have a combined limit on out-of-pocket costs of $10,000 or less, though this averaged $8,818 in 2019.[30]

Competition among MA plans has historically fueled the inclusion of various supplemental services not covered under traditional Medicare. For example, in 1986, a survey of Medicare HMO beneficiaries revealed that 84.7 percent had prescription drug coverage,[31] a benefit added to the traditional Medicare program by Congress 17 years later.

Private-sector innovation has allowed for health plans to experiment with new benefits, evaluating both satisfaction and cost-effectiveness while focusing on functional areas core to independence. The story here is similar to prescription drugs, with research from 2016 demonstrating that an estimated 62 percent of MA beneficiaries had dental benefits while 67 percent had vision benefits. In contrast, among beneficiaries enrolled in traditional Medicare, 96 percent lacked vision insurance and 79 percent lacked dental coverage.[32]

Plans continue to experiment with other supplemental benefits, such as wheelchair ramps, bathroom grab bars, meal delivery after hospital discharge, home modifications, gym memberships, and even the Apple Watch.[33] Flexibility is key, helping elderly and disabled Americans maintain their independence.[34] In contrast, innovation is challenging in traditional Medicare, which requires rulemaking and frequent statutory change to redefine or expand benefit categories. Beneficiaries cover the gap, with 8 in 10 beneficiaries possessing some form of supplemental insurance (e.g., aptly named Medigap policies, employer-sponsored insurance, or even Medicaid).[35]

Coordinated and integrated care, largely unavailable in FFS Medicare, presents another potential boon for beneficiaries. Research on MA has demonstrated benefits, including less intense post-acute care use,[36] lower readmission and preventable hospital rates,[37] more appropriate health care utilization,[38] and decreased intensive care unit use,[39] to name a few. While researchers debate the exact benefits, MA offers the potential for integrated care, a challenge in the FFS system.

Finally, vulnerable populations—such as those living in institutions or those with both Medicare and Medicaid—face even greater challenges in managing their care and health. More than half live with at least one functional impairment in activities of daily living[40] and are almost twice as likely to self-report their health to be "fair" or "poor" when compared to other Medicare beneficiaries.[41] MA provides special flexibility for these and other groups, allowing for benefit customization in the form of SNPs. Auto-enrollment would simplify the organization and coordination of health benefits for disadvantaged populations.

In exchange for limitations on their financial liability and for obtaining supplemental benefits, beneficiaries are subject to some utilization and access controls. A network of providers is common among MA plans and often where concerns over the program are directed. Yet a 2017 analysis found 65 percent of enrollees to be in plans featuring either "medium" (accepted by 30 percent to 69 percent of physicians in an average county) or "broad" (70 percent or more) networks.[42] Consistent with this, almost two-thirds of MA participants are enrolled in HMO plans and the remainder in PPO plans.[43] Given beneficiary experience with employer-sponsored insurance,[44] the trade-offs between greater benefits and utilization and access controls are familiar to consumers. Consumers have voted with their feet and are leaving traditional Medicare for Medicare Advantage. In 2020, the FFS Medicare program, experiencing a steady annual decline since 2010, covered 60 percent of beneficiaries.[45]

Medicare Advantage: A Natural Experiment in Health Plan Competition

Under MA, policymakers have set up a natural experiment in health plan competition.[46] The CMS contracts with insurance companies and integrated delivery systems to design and administer health insurance plans that must meet or exceed the coverage standards of traditional Medicare. A rate filing or bid process takes place in which the CMS agrees to pay plans a fixed monthly amount per beneficiary, a method known as capitation. Capitation rates are risk adjusted[47] based on each beneficiaries' health and eligibility statuses to best account for the total predicted future cost of their care. Health plans then assume risk and responsibility for making payment arrangements with providers and designing and administrating benefit packages for beneficiaries.

The opportunity for comprehensive quality improvement lies in the ability of MA plans to operate outside the FFS model, using this flexibility to distribute risk in more ways that both increase physician accountability and incentivize value (see fig. 6.3.) As previously described, there are a number of payment arrangements these plans and providers can enter (gainsharing, risk corridors, partial capitation, private FFS, and episode bundling,[48] among others), all of which have strengths and weaknesses in generating more value for the dollar.[49] With 41 percent of MA spending directed through risk-transfer payment models, MA exceeds other plan markets in transferring risk to providers.

With the ability to be thoughtful in how providers are paid for services, private plans have the tools to reduce the delivery system's focus on intensity and volume of care regulation. Further, a capitated

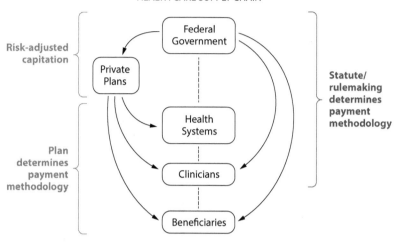

In **Medicare Advantage**, the federal government capitates plans. Plans have flexibility in how to distribute and pay for risk throughout the supply chain.

Fee-for-Service Medicare has statutory payment methodologies, while administrative price setting is executed by annual rulemaking.

HEALTH CARE SUPPLY CHAIN

Risk-adjusted capitation

Federal Government

Private Plans

Statute/ rulemaking determines payment methodology

Health Systems

Plan determines payment methodology

Clinicians

Beneficiaries

FIGURE 6.3. Medicare Advantage vs. Fee-for-Service Medicare. *Source:* Brian J. Miller, "Regulation & Principles of Health Insurance," lecture at Kenan-Flagler Business School on April 12, 2019.

model incentivizes and empowers providers to steer consumers to appropriate care, be it in the form of increased rates of bypass surgery for patients with cardiac disease, lower utilization of emergency rooms,[50] or greater utilization of preventive and screening services.[51] MA plans may also tier providers, grading providers on performance. Additional cost savings are available to beneficiaries for receiving care from top-tier providers, making tiered networks a tool for steering both consumer and provider behavior toward value.[52]

Responsive to the needs of beneficiaries and concerns raised by researchers, policymakers have continued to innovate Medicare Advantage program design. Historically, researchers have noted that plans preferentially enrolled healthy beneficiaries while higher-cost beneficiaries disenrolled, choosing to elect fee-for-service.[53] The Medicare Modernization Act responded with special needs plans, targeting high-cost beneficiaries with better benefits customization. Further iterations in payment methodology have helped eliminate inappropriate overpayment of plans, with recent research noting that Medicare Advantage payments to hospitals are equivalent[54] to or lower[55] than those in the fee-for-service program. Overall spending in Medicare Advantage demonstrates both regional variation[56] and marginally lower costs[57] and is associated with positive spillover effects in fee-for-service, decreasing county-level per capita fee-for-service expenditures as Medicare Advantage penetration increases.[58]

A defined budget for MA plans—based upon risk-adjusted capitation—facilitates budgetary planning on the part of policymakers and provides the CMS a more flexible tool to shape health insurance markets. In contrast, Medicare FFS, deploying administrative price setting without downstream utilization controls, leaves its payer—the CMS—with few mechanisms to budget for or manage health care expenditures on a large scale.

What's Next? Lessons from Retirement Planning

Congress should change the default auto-assignment from traditional Medicare to Medicare Advantage, a reform advantageous to both beneficiaries and policymakers who desire budgetary planning. Currently, new enrollees are defaulted into traditional Medicare (with penalties for late enrollment), with MA participation requiring an elective, opt-in process. Under today's model, about 29 percent of new beneficiaries choose to enroll in MA annually,[59] an increase from 22 percent in 2011.[60] In this new model, newly eligible beneficiaries would—by default—be automatically enrolled in MA, with a defined period to change plans or disenroll and elect traditional Medicare should they wish to do so. Plans and programs in both Alabama and New Jersey have already begun exclusively directing coverage of retirees' benefits to MA plans, resulting in state enrollment increases of 90,000 and 60,000 beneficiaries, respectively, over a single enrollment period.[61]

Similar enrollment arrangements in other consumer marketplaces have seen dramatic success in raising participation rates. Long proposed by policy experts,[62] retirement plan adoption of automatic enrollment policies drove significant increases in employee participation from 2003 to 2017. By 2017, 63 percent of new plan entrants joined via auto-enrollment, according to plan data from the Vanguard Group, a leading company in 401(k) and defined contribution retirement savings plans. By 2018, plans with an automatic enrollment feature—requiring those not interested to opt out—had a 92 percent participation rate, while those with voluntary opt-in enrollment saw a participation rate of only 57 percent,[63] a finding replicated in academic research regarding 401(k) participation by workers across industries.[64]

While the principles of auto-enrollment for retirement are applicable, auto-enrollment in health plan products merits special considerations, as access to health care and pharmaceuticals, choice of physicians, and obtaining hospital and emergency care when needed is sharply distinct from the economic problem of saving for retirement. Health—and health care—affects one's ability to function in the world and is an intensely personal and important choice. Health care utilization, as opposed to retirement costs, is more varied and challenging to predict due to its numerous inputs, including the natural and constructed environment, individual choices, genetics, occupation, and other factors. Health insurance literacy, a well-recognized problem,[65] presents further consumer protection challenges to be surmounted.

The Next Generation of Medicare Reform: Changing Default Enrollment

Most individuals find themselves eligible for Medicare when they turn 65 years old and either are required to activate and pay premiums for Part A hospital coverage or, if they have already received Social Security benefits for four months, are automatically enrolled in premium-free Part A coverage.[66] Consumers automatically enrolled in Part A are secondarily auto-enrolled in Medicare Part B, while those paying Part A premiums have to elect Part B coverage and pay premiums.[67]

Under the proposal to initiate default assignment into MA plans, the pool of individuals newly eligible for Medicare benefits would go unchanged. If new beneficiaries did not select an MA plan or elect FFS Medicare, they would be automatically assigned to an MA plan. This policy change would affect only those who become newly eligible, not those already receiving Medicare coverage. Beneficiaries would retain the ability to delay their Medicare Part B eligibility while continuing commercial coverage through their employers. Default assignment into MA would be initiated upon Part B election or Medicare auto-enrollment if eligible for Social Security. Newly eligible beneficiaries of the multiple populations that make up the Medicare program would be subject to auto-assignment, while special populations, such as dual-eligibles, would be auto-enrolled in the appropriate special needs plan.

We suggest auto-assignment be an option exclusive to MA plans with a star rating of 3.5 or higher,[68] protecting beneficiaries from lower-quality plans while also not overly anchoring the market in favor of incumbent plans. To facilitate this policy change, health plans electing and eligible to participate in auto-assignment would be required to offer at least one zero-premium,[69] basic coverage plan providing minimum Part A, B, and D benefits. These requirements would level the playing field among the health plans competing for the same beneficiaries, with the January to March open-enrollment period providing beneficiaries an opportunity to change plans. Additional criteria would need to be defined to ensure that beneficiary preferences, including provider choice, would be appropriately factored into the assignment process.[70] Finally, beneficiaries who remain unsatisfied with the available choices in the MA marketplace would be able to disenroll into FFS during the existing standard annual disenrollment period from January 1 through February 14.

Several health insurance markets support this precedent. In states such as New Mexico and New York, Medicaid beneficiaries who become newly eligible for Medicare are auto-assigned to dual-eligible special needs plans (D-SNPs), which have customized benefits for dual-eligibles. Other beneficiaries with preexisting commercial coverage can be auto-assigned to a like-plan product (e.g., HMO to HMO or PPO to PPO) within the same parent organization, ensuring preservation of their existing provider relationships. Managed Medicaid markets also deploy auto-assignment to promote both a relationship with a primary care physician and a managed care plan, providing lessons for the MA marketplace.[71] For example, Nebraska's managed Medicaid program, Heritage Health, utilizes equitable auto-assignment, preserves primary care physician relationships, and additionally combats health insurance literacy challenges by preferentially auto-enrolling members in the same plan if a household member is already enrolled.[72]

Policymakers have multiple routes for implementation. CMS Innovation Center waiver authority (Section 3021 of the ACA) would facilitate modification of the enrollment process and creation of an innovation center model with a population targeting all Medicare beneficiaries. Alternatively, Congress could enact statutory change, tying auto-enrollment in MA to the Part A auto-enrollment and Part B benefit-election processes.

Consequences of implementation are varied. Beneficiaries would gain greater financial protections along with supplementation benefits in exchange for some network access and utilization controls while still retaining the ability to elect into FFS. Uniform access to supplemental benefits would promote health plan innovation in benefit design. Health plans would gain market share in the Medicare marketplace due to auto-enrollment, further incentivizing development of care management programs. It would broaden the actuarial risk pool, as the vast majority of new Medicare beneficiaries would be enrolled in MA.[73] Policymakers would obtain improved budgetary forecasting[74] and new levers for budgetary control, as auto-enrollment would increase the penetration of risk-adjusted, capitated plan products in the Medicare marketplace. Thus, the focus of Congress and the

CMS would shift to modifying future spending and adjusting capitation rates and risk adjustment methodologies as opposed to administrative price setting of individual services as exists in FFS. Furthermore, by increasing the use of MA, policymakers would continue the healthy shift of medical necessity, formulary design, and benefits design to health plans, continuing to shift the CMS from its role as a FFS health plan operator to a market regulator.

Even without this change, participation in Medicare Advantage has more than doubled over the past decade. In 2020, two in five Medicare beneficiaries, comprising over 23 million individuals, enrolled in an MA plan. The Congressional Budget Office now projects that 47 percent of Medicare beneficiaries will get their coverage from MA plans by 2029, noting that the program grew 71 percent since the passage of the ACA.[75] The growth of MA emphasizes the need for policy innovation and subsequent statutory change in other areas of program design, such as MA's bidding system, which is anchored in FFS benchmarks.[76]

Looking Ahead

The transition to value in the health care system necessitates comprehensive changes in the way care is financed and delivered. Enacting statutory change to allow auto-assignment of beneficiaries into MA plans marks the next step on the path to value. Doing so would provide policymakers with better levers for spending control while facilitating value-based development and innovation in supplemental benefit design, helping taxpayers and beneficiaries alike. Finally, by fixing financing first, policymakers can facilitate the transition of the largest health plan market—the Medicare program—to a defined contribution by way of a risk-adjusted, capitated financing model.

Medicare Advantage is a market-tested, federally protected, and innovative marketplace with the potential to provide better health care. It is up to Congress to deploy it to its full potential.

• •

BRIAN J. MILLER, MD, MBA, MPH, is a hospitalist and public health physician who serves as an assistant professor of medicine and business (courtesy) at Johns Hopkins University and Nonresident Fellow at the American Enterprise Institute. GAIL R. WILENSKY, PHD, is a Senior Fellow at Project Hope and a former administrator at the Centers for Medicare and Medicaid Services. The authors are grateful for and would like to acknowledge Jennifer M. Slota for her research and editorial assistance.

NOTES

1. Juliette Cubanski, Tricia Neuman, and Meredith Freed, "The Facts on Medicare Spending and Financing," Kaiser Family Foundation, August 20, 2019, https://files.kff .org/attachment/Issue-Brief-Facts-on-Medicaid-Spending-and-Financing.

2. US Census Bureau, "Older People Projected to Outnumber Children for First Time in US History," March 13, 2018, https://www.census.gov/newsroom/press -releases/2018/cb18-41-population-projections.html.

3. This is an estimate for 2023. Boards of Trustees of the Federal Hospital Insurance and the Supplementary Medical Insurance Trust Funds, *2022 Annual Report of the Boards of Trustees* (Washington, DC: Centers for Medicare and Medicaid Services, June 2, 2022), 181, table V.B3, https://www.cms.gov/files /document/2022-medicare-trustees-report.pdf.

4. Ezekiel J. Emanuel, "Democrats Are Having the Wrong Health Care Debate," *New York Times*, August 2, 2019, https://www.nytimes.com/2019/08/02/opinion /democrats-health-care.html.

5. Robert E. Moffit and Alyene Senger, "Medicare's Rising Costs—and the Urgent Need for Reform," Backgrounder no. 2779 (Washington, DC: The Heritage Foundation, March 22, 2013), https://www.heritage.org/health-care-reform /report/medicares-rising-costs-and-the-urgent-need-reform.

6. Congressional Budget Office, *The 2019 Long-Term Budget Outlook* (Washington, DC: Congressional Budget Office, June 2019), https://www.cbo.gov/system /files/2019-06/55331-LTBO-2.pdf.

7. US Department of Health and Human Services, Centers for Disease Control and Prevention, "Mortality Trends in the United States, 1900–2018," updated August 25, 2020, https://www.cdc.gov/nchs/data-visualization/mortality-trends /index.htm.

8. Intensity of care is determined jointly by patients and physicians. Consider an otherwise healthy 35-year-old man with no comorbidities presenting to the physician in clinic with burning chest discomfort after eating. A reasonable clinical strategy would be to have the patient try a six-week prescribed course of a stomach acid–suppressing medication to empirically treat reflux, returning if the symptoms persist or there is lack of improvement. An alternative, high-intensity strategy would be to simultaneously conduct a screening electrocardiogram and echocardiogram to assess for arrhythmias and heart failure, respectively.

9. FFS prices also anchor components of the MA program. For example, plans must pay out-of-network physicians the lesser of billed charge or the Medicare fee schedule. See Centers for Medicare and Medicaid Services (CMS), *MA Payment Guide for Out of Network Payment* (Baltimore: CMS, April 15, 2015), https://www .cms.gov/Medicare/Health-Plans/MedicareAdvtgSpecRateStats/Downloads /OONPayments.pdf.

10. From 1967 to 1983, utilization of physician and outpatient services per beneficiary doubled, while the annual compound real rate of growth was 9.1 percent for the period 1967–1984. See Marian Gornick, Jay N. Greenberg, Paul W. Eggers, and Allen Dobson, "Twenty Years of Medicare and Medicaid: Covered Populations, Use of Benefits, and Program Expenditures," *Health Care Financing Review*, annual supplement (December 1985): 13–59.

11. John K. Inglehart, "Medicare Begins Prospective Payment of Hospitals," *New England Journal of Medicine* 308, no. 23 (1983): 1428–32.

12. "Medicare Payment Systems, What's Changed: Acute Care Hospital Inpatient Prospective Payment System," CMS Medicare Learning Network, February 2022, https://www.cms.gov/Outreach-and-Education/Medicare -Learning-Network-MLN/MLNProducts/html/medicare-payment-systems.html.

13. MedPAC, *Hospital Acute Inpatient Services Payment System* (Washington, DC: Medicare Payment Advisory Commission, November 2021), https://www.medpac .gov/wp-content/uploads/2021/11/medpac_payment_basics_21_hospital_final _sec.pdf.

14. MedPAC, *Hospice Services Payment System* (Washington, DC: Medicare Payment Advisory Commission, November 2021), https://www.medpac.gov/wp -content/uploads/2021/11/medpac_payment_basics_21_hospice_final_sec.pdf.

15. MedPAC, *Home Health Services Payment System* (Washington, DC: Medicare Payment Advisory Commission, October 2021), https://www.medpac.gov/wp -content/uploads/2021/11/medpac_payment_basics_21_hha_final_sec.pdf.

16. MedPAC, *Outpatient Hospital Services Payment System* (Washington, DC: Medicare Payment Advisory Commission, November 2021), https://www.medpac .gov/wp-content/uploads/2021/11/medpac_payment_basics_21_opd_final_sec .pdf.

17. Previous technical attempts to more accurately price physician services in the Medicare program have had a challenging history. For example, a failed attempt to control Part B spending was executed as part of the Omnibus Budget Reconciliation Act of 1989, which created the resource-based relative value scale, which has long been subject to mispricing and lobbying. See Paul B. Ginsburg and Robert A. Berenson, "Revising Medicare's Physician Fee Schedule—Much Activity, Little Change," *New England Journal of Medicine* 356, no. 12 (2007): 1201–2.

18. CMS, "Final Rule Medicare Program; CY 2020 Revisions to the Payment Policy Under the Physician Fee Schedule," Federal Register 84 (November 15, 2019), 62568–63563.

19. "CMS Releases Final 2018 QPP Performance Results: Max Positive 2020 Payment Adjustment Is 1.68%," Society for Post-Acute and Long-Term Care

Medicine, January 9, 2020, https://paltc.org/publications/cms-releases-final-2018
-qpp-performance-results-max-positive-2020-payment-adjustment.

20. Boards of Trustees of the Federal Hospital Insurance and the Supplementary Medical Insurance Trust Funds, *2020 Annual Report of the Boards of Trustees* (Washington, DC: Centers for Medicare and Medicaid Services, April 22, 2020), https://www.cms.gov/files/document/2020-medicare-trustees-report.pdf.

21. Medicare is statutorily limited in the amount against which a provider can balance bill a patient to 115 percent of the Medicare physician fee schedule. See Cristina Boccuti, "Pay a Visit to the Doctor: Current Financial Protections for Medicare Patients When Receiving Physician Services," Kaiser Family Foundation, November 2016, http://files.kff.org/attachment/Issue-Brief-Paying-a-Visit-to-the -Doctor-Current-Financial-Protections.

22. The HMO Act of 1973 required employers with 25 or more employees offering private health insurance to offer an HMO option.

23. Yash M. Patel and Stuart Guterman, "The Evolution of Private Plans in Medicare," Commonwealth Fund, December 8, 2017, https://www.common wealthfund.org/publications/issue-briefs/2017/dec/evolution-private-plans -medicare.

24. CMS, "Milestones 1937–2015," July 2015, https://www.cms.gov/About -CMS-Agency-Information/History/Downloads/Medicare-and-Medicaid -Milestones-1937-2015.pdf.

25. Carlo Zarabozo and Scott Harrison, "Payment Policy and the Growth of Medicare Advantage," *Health Affairs* 27, supplement 1 (2008): w55–w67.

26. Lisa Sprague, "The Star Rating System and Medicare Advantage Plans," NHPF Issue Brief no. 854 (Washington, DC: National Health Policy Forum, May 5, 2015); Dan Jamieson, Monisha Machado-Pereira, Stephanie Carlton, and Cara Repasky, "Assessing the Medicare Advantage Star Ratings," McKinsey & Company Healthcare Systems & Services, July 31, 2018, https://www.mckinsey.com/industries /healthcare-systems-and-services/our-insights/assessing-the-medicare-advantage -stars-ratings.

27. CMS, "Medicare Advantage Premiums Continue to Decline While Plan Choices and Benefits Increase in 2019," September 28, 2018, https://www.cms.gov /newsroom/press-releases/medicare-advantage-premiums-continue-decline-while -plan-choices-and-benefits-increase-2019.

28. Gretchen Jacobson, Meredith Freed, Anthony Damico, and Tricia Neuman, "A Dozen Facts about Medicare Advantage in 2019," Kaiser Family Foundation, June 6, 2019, https://www.kff.org/medicare/issue-brief/a-dozen-facts-about -medicare-advantage-in-2019.

29. CMS, "Trump Administration Drives Down Medicare Advantage and Part D Premiums for Seniors," September 24, 2019, https://www.cms.gov/newsroom /press-releases/trump-administration-drives-down-medicare-advantage-and-part -d-premiums-seniors.

30. Jacobson et al., "A Dozen Facts about Medicare Advantage in 2019."

31. Alma McMillan, James Lubitz, and Delores Russell, "Medicare Enrollment in Health Maintenance Organizations," *Health Care Financing Review* 8, no. 3 (1987): 87–93.

32. Amber Willink, Nicholas S. Reed, Bonnielin Swenor, Leah Leinbach, Eva H. DuGoff, and Karen Davis, "Dental, Vision, and Hearing Services: Access, Spending, and Coverage for Medicare Beneficiaries," *Health Affairs* 39, no. 2 (2020): 297–304.

33. Christina Farr, "Private Medicare Plan Devoted Health Says It Is the First to Cover Apple Watch as a Benefit," CNBC, October 7, 2019, https://www.cnbc.com /2019/10/07/devoted-medicare-advantage-plan-covering-apple-watch-as-a-benefit .html.

34. Alison Silvers, Torrie Fields, Anna Kytonen, and Diane E. Meier, "Medicare Advantage Flexibility: Improving Care for Seriously Ill Beneficiaries," *Health Affairs Blog*, July 6, 2018, https://www.healthaffairs.org/do/10.1377/hblog20180702 .641853/full.

35. Juliette Cubanski, Anthony Damico, Tricia Neuman, and Gretchen Jacobson, "Sources of Supplemental Coverage among Medicare Beneficiaries in 2016," Kaiser Family Foundation, November 28, 2018, https://www.kff.org /medicare/issue-brief/sources-of-supplemental-coverage-among-medicare -beneficiaries-in-2016.

36. Peter J. Huckfeldt, José J. Escarce, Brendan Rabideau, Pinar Karaca-Mandic, and Neeraj Sood, "Less Intense Postacute Care, Better Outcomes for Enrollees in Medicare Advantage than Those in Fee-for-Service," *Health Affairs* 36, no. 1 (2017): 91–100.

37. Gerard Anderson, *The Benefits of Care Coordination: Comparison of Medicare Fee-for-Service and Medicare Advantage* (Baltimore: Johns Hopkins University, Center for Hospital Finance and Management, September 1, 2009), https:// citeseerx.ist.psu.edu/viewdoc/download?doi=10.1.1.597.645&rep=rep1&type =pdf.

38. Bruce E. Landon, Alan M. Zaslavsky, Robert C. Saunders, L. Gregory Pawlson, Joseph P. Newhouse, and John Z. Ayanian, "Analysis of Medicare Advantage HMOs Compared with Traditional Medicare Shows Lower Use of Many Services During 2003–2009," *Health Affairs* 31, no. 12 (2012): 2609–17.

39. David J. Meyers, Vincent Mor, and Momotazur Rahman, "Provider Integrated Medicare Advantage Plans Are Associated with Differences in Patterns of Inpatient Care," *Health Affairs* 39, no. 5 (2020): 843–51.

40. "Activities of daily living" describe basic skills required to care independently for oneself, such as eating, bathing, toileting, and mobility. See Peter F. Edemekong, Deb L. Bomgaars, Sukesh Sukumaran, and Shoshana B. Levy, "Activities of Daily Living," in *StatPearls* [online] (Treasure Island, FL: StatPearls Publishing), updated September 26, 2021, https://www.ncbi.nlm.nih.gov/books/NBK470404.

41. Juliette Cubanski, Christina Swoope, Cristina Boccuti, Gretchen Jacobson, Giselle Casillas, Shannon Griffin, and Tricia Neuman, "A Primer on Medicare: Key Facts about the Medicare Program and the People It Covers," Kaiser Family

Foundation, March 20, 2015, https://www.kff.org/report-section/a-primer-on-medicare-what-is-the-role-of-medicare-for-dual-eligible-beneficiaries.

42. Gretchen Jacobson, Matthew Rae, Tricia Neuman, Kendal Orgera, and Cristina Boccuti, "Medicare Advantage: How Robust Are Plans' Physician Networks?," Kaiser Family Foundation, October 5, 2017, https://www.kff.org/medicare/report/medicare-advantage-how-robust-are-plans-physician-networks.

43. "Medicare Advantage," Kaiser Family Foundation, June 6, 2019, https://www.kff.org/medicare/fact-sheet/medicare-advantage.

44. "2019 Employer Health Benefits Survey," Kaiser Family Foundation, September 25, 2019, https://www.kff.org/report-section/ehbs-2019-summary-of-findings.

45. In June 2020, 24.97 million out of 62.50 million Medicare beneficiaries were enrolled in an MA plan (see "Medicare Monthly Enrollment," Data.CMS.gov, last updated March 2022, https://www.cms.gov/Research-Statistics-Data-and-Systems/Statistics-Trends-and-Reports/Dashboard/Medicare-Enrollment/Enrollment%20Dashboard.html).

46. Plan competition is constrained as plans bid against a benchmark equal to the average FFS spending per capita in the county as opposed to competing against other plans. Discussion of how to improve the competitive bidding system is both a worthy and separate topic that is outside the scope of this chapter.

47. MedPAC has noted the need for further refinement of CMS risk adjustment methodology. See MedPAC, "The Medicare Advantage Program: Status Report," chapter 12 in *March 2021 Report to the Congress: Medicare Payment Policy* (Washington, DC: Medicare Payment Advisory Commission, 2021), 353–95, https://www.medpac.gov/wp-content/uploads/import_data/scrape_files/docs/default-source/reports/mar21_medpac_report_to_the_congress_sec.pdf.

48. Michael L. Barnett, Andrew Wilcock, J. Michael McWilliams, Arnold M. Epstein, Karen E. Joynt Maddox, E. John Orav, David C. Grabowski, and Ateev Mehrotra, "Two-Year Evaluation of Mandatory Bundled Payments for Joint Replacement," *New England Journal of Medicine* 380, no. 3 (2019): 252–62.

49. Robert A. Berenson, Divvy K. Upadhyay, Suzanne F. Delbanco, and Roslyn Murray, *Payment Methods and Benefit Designs: How They Work and How They Work Together to Improve Health Care* (Washington, DC: Urban Institute, updated June 10, 2016), https://www.urban.org/sites/default/files/publication/80301/2000776-Payment-Methods-How-They-Work.pdf.

50. Brandon E. Landon, Alan M. Zaslavsky, Robert C. Saunders, L. Gregory Pawlson, Joseph P. Newhouse, and John Z. Ayanian, "Analysis of Medicare Advantage HMOs Compared with Traditional Medicare Shows Lower Use of Many Services During 2003–09," *Health Affairs* 31, no. 12 (2012): 2609–17; Avalere Health, "Medicare Advantage Achieves Cost-Effective Care and Better Outcomes for Beneficiaries with Chronic Conditions Relative to Fee-for-Service Medicare," press release, July 11, 2018, https://avalere.com/press-releases/medicare-advantage-achieves-better-health-outcomes-and-lower-utilization-of-high-cost-services-compared-to-fee-for-service-medicare.

51. John Z. Ayanian, Bruce E. Landon, Alan M. Zaslavsky, Robert C. Saunders, L. Gregory Pawlson, and Joseph P. Newhouse, "Medicare Beneficiaries More Likely to Receive Appropriate Ambulatory Services in HMOs than in Traditional Medicare," *Health Affairs* 32, no. 7 (2013): 1228–35.

52. Stephanie Kanwit, "Provider Networks in the Medicare Advantage Program," at hearing before the Senate Special Committee on Aging, *Medicare Advantage: Changing Networks and Effects on Consumers*, 113th Congress, January 2014, https://www.aging.senate.gov/download/stephanie-kanwit.

53. Momotazur Rahman, Laura Keohane, Amal N. Trivedi, and Vincent Mor, "High-Cost Patients Had Substantial Rates of Leaving Medicare Advantage and Joining Traditional Medicare," *Health Affairs* 34, no. 10 (2015): 1675–81; Claire K. Ankuda, Katherine A. Ornstein, Kenneth E. Covinsky, Evan Bollens-Lund, Diane E. Meier, and Amy S. Kelley, "Switching between Medicare Advantage and Traditional Medicare Before and After the Onset of Functional Disability," *Health Affairs* 39, no. 5 (2020): 809–18.

54. Robert A. Berenson, Jonathan H. Sunshine, David Helms, and Emily Lawton, "Why Medicare Advantage Plans Pay Hospitals Traditional Medicare Prices," *Health Affairs* 34, no. 8 (2015): 1289–95.

55. Laurence C. Baker, M. Kate Bundorf, Aileen M. Devlin, and Daniel P. Kessler, "Medicare Advantage Plans Pay Hospitals Less Than Traditional Medicare Pays," *Health Affairs* 35, no. 8 (2016): 1444–51.

56. Brian Biles, Giselle Casillas, and Stuart Guterman, "Does Medicare Advantage Cost Less Than Traditional Medicare?," The Commonwealth Fund, January 28, 2016, https://www.commonwealthfund.org/publications/issue-briefs/2016/jan/does-medicare-advantage-cost-less-traditional-medicare.

57. Vilsa Curto, Liran Einav, Amy Finkelstein, Jonathan Levin, and Jay Bhattacharya, "Health Care Spending and Utilization in Public and Private Medicare," *American Economic Journal: Applied Economics* 11, no. 2 (2019): 302–32.

58. Garret Johnson, José F. Figueroa, Xiner Zhou, E. John Orav, and Ashish K. Jha, "Recent Growth in Medicare Advantage Enrollment Associated with Decreased Fee-for-Service Spending in Certain US Counties," *Health Affairs* 35, no. 9 (2016): 1707–15.

59. Gretchen Jacobson, Tricia Neuman, Meredith Freed, and Anthony Damico, "What Percent of New Medicare Beneficiaries Are Enrolling in Medicare Advantage?," Kaiser Family Foundation, June 6, 2019, https://www.kff.org/medicare/issue-brief/what-percent-of-new-medicare-beneficiaries-are-enrolling-in-medicare-advantage.

60. Gretchen A. Jacobson, Patricia Neuman, and Anthony Damico, "At Least Half of New Medicare Advantage Enrollees Had Switched from Traditional Medicare during 2006–11," *Health Affairs* 34, no. 1 (2015): 48–55.

61. Gretchen Jacobson, Anthony Damico, Tricia Neuman, and Marsha Gold, "Medicare Advantage 2017 Spotlight: Enrollment Market Update," Kaiser Family Foundation, June 6, 2017, https://www.kff.org/medicare/issue-brief/medicare-advantage-2017-spotlight-enrollment-market-update.

62. John Scott and Andrew Blevins, "Automatic Enrollment Can Boost Retirement Plan Participation," Pew Charitable Trusts, August 15, 2018, https://www.pewtrusts.org/en/research-and-analysis/articles/2018/08/15/automatic-enrollment-can-boost-retirement-plan-participation.

63. "How America Saves 2018," Vanguard, June 2018, https://alaska.shrm.org/sites/alaska.shrm.org/files/How%20America%20Saves%20Vanguard%202018.pdf.

64. James J. Choi, David Laibson, Brigitte C. Madrian, and Andrew Metrick, "Defined Contribution Pensions: Plan Rules, Participant Decisions, and the Path of Least Resistance," NBER Working Paper no. 8655 (Cambridge, MA: National Bureau of Economic Research, December 2001), https://www.nber.org/papers/w8655.pdf.

65. Mira Norton, Liz Hamel, and Mollyann Brodie, "Assessing American's Familiarity with Health Insurance Terms and Concepts," Kaiser Family Foundation, November 11, 2014, https://www.kff.org/health-reform/poll-finding/assessing-americans-familiarity-with-health-insurance-terms-and-concepts.

66. CMS, "Original Medicare (Part A and B) Eligibility and Enrollment," updated December 1, 2021, https://www.cms.gov/Medicare/Eligibility-and-Enrollment/OrigMedicarePartABEligEnrol.

67. Individuals who delay or forgo Medicare coverage will face lifetime late penalties added to their premiums upon eventual enrollment for every year prior that they were not enrolled. The enrollment period begins three months before the individual's birthday month and ends three months following it.

68. To facilitate informed, optimal decision-making by beneficiaries, the CMS closely evaluates the quality of MA plans annually via the Star Rating system. Plans are awarded one to five stars based on their performance across five categories: preventive services access, management of chronic conditions, overall member experience and satisfaction, frequency of complaints and disenrollment, and customer service quality. The CMS projected that over 81 percent of MA beneficiaries would be enrolled in plans rated four stars or higher in 2020, a milestone met in 2021. See "Trump Administration Drives Access to More High-Quality Medicare Plan Choices in 2020," CMS Newsroom, October 11, 2019, https://www.cms.gov/newsroom/press-releases/trump-administration-drives-access-more-high-quality-medicare-plan-choices-2020; Jeannie Fuglesten Biniek, Meredith Freed, Anthony Damico, and Tricia Neuman, "Medicare Advantage in 2021: Star Ratings and Bonuses," Kaiser Family Foundation, June 21, 2021, https://www.kff.org/medicare/issue-brief/medicare-advantage-in-2021-star-ratings-and-bonuses. The Star Rating program is an initial attempt at grading plan quality; further modernization is needed, a topic outside the scope of this chapter. Our intent in recommending Congress use the Star Rating program as part of an auto-assignment methodology is to protect beneficiaries, as plans with three or fewer stars are at risk of losing their MA contracts while setting a bar of four stars or higher could anchor the market in favor of incumbent plans. Auto-

assignment would have an additional upside of encouraging companies to enter the markets where there is limited plan competition today.

69. If a beneficiary did not select an MA plan or elect FFS, auto-assignment into a zero-premium plan would ensure that he or she is not automatically obligated for further out-of-pocket expenses. To some degree, this will anchor auto-assignment into "moderate breadth" HMO and PPO plans. Beneficiaries will still retain the option of selecting their own plans, changing plans, or electing into FFS, which may have broader networks.

70. Previous provider choices by beneficiaries should be respected as part of the auto-assignment. For example, where possible, a beneficiary who undergoes auto-assignment into a zero-premium, 3.5-star or higher MA plan should preferentially be placed in a plan where their primary care physician (if they have a preexisting relationship with one) is in network and on a preferred tier.

71. Consider the example of a husband and wife, where the husband is retired and already enrolled in a Kaiser Permanente MA HMO plan. His wife subsequently retires and is eligible for Medicare. She can either select an MA plan, elect into FFS, or decline to make a decision. If the latter, she is defaulted into MA and subject to auto-assignment. Auto-assignment would place her in a zero-premium, 3.5-star or higher plan and would preferentially place her in a Kaiser Permanente MA HMO plan, "piggybacking" off any preexisting household knowledge of health benefits.

72. See page 34 of the "Request for Proposal for Contractual Services Form," Solicitation no. RFP 5151 Z1, October 21, 2015, State of Nebraska, available at https://openminds.com/wp-content/uploads/rfp/102215h.pdf.

73. Coupling auto-enrollment with default assignment into MA would address historical concerns voiced by health policy experts regarding favorable plan selection of healthy beneficiaries, as new beneficiaries would default into an MA plan.

74. Administrative price setting in traditional FFS Medicare, as opposed to MA's risk-adjusted, capitated model, has created difficulties in forecasting expenditures. Economists' projections of Part A and Part B expenditures made in the 1970s and 1980s were notoriously inaccurate when compared with actual expenditures. See Mark Freeland, George Calat, and Carol Ellen Schendler, "Projections of National Health Expenditures, 1980, 1985, and 1990," *Health Care Financing Review* 1, no. 3 (1980): 1–27; Rabah Kamal, Daniel McDermott, Gioriando Ramirez, and Cynthia Cox, "How Has US Spending on Healthcare Changed Over Time?," Kaiser Family Foundation, December 23, 2020, https://www.healthsystemtracker.org/chart-collection/u-s-spending-healthcare-changed-time.

75. Jacobson et al. "Medicare Advantage 2017 Spotlight: Enrollment Market Update."

76. See Section 1853 of the Social Security Act, 42 U.S.C. 1395w-23, accessed September 9, 2020, https://uscode.house.gov/view.xhtml?req=(title:42%20 section:1395w-23%20edition:prelim).

PART III

TRANSITIONING TO PREMIUM SUPPORT
The Promise of Greater Personal Choice and Market Competition

Medicare Advantage's record suggests it can be leveraged to make structural reforms to traditional Medicare that deliver even greater value. To argue this point, Robert Emmet Moffit, PhD, starts with outlining how Medicare Advantage can serve, if further improved, as the platform for a model where dollars follow patients in the form of "premium support," a defined contribution system that allows beneficiaries to direct their government subsidies to plans of their choosing (chapter 7). Such a system would empower beneficiaries to choose the coverage that they determine is best for them.

For such a reform to succeed, policymakers must also pursue structural changes to both Medicare and Medicare Advantage that build on what's working today. Joseph R. Antos, PhD, explains the need to modernize the traditional program so that it offers standard, more attractive benefits to enrollees (chapter 8). Edmund F. Haislmaier details needed changes to risk adjustment for both traditional Medicare and private health plans with the goal of defining market conditions so that plans compete to cover high-risk patients (chapter 9). Prescription drug coverage in Medicare today uses a form of premium support, and Doug Badger draws lessons from that experience about what works well and what could be improved both within that program and as part of structural changes to broader Medicare (chapter 10).

Policymakers seeking to advance these reforms could also look to the bipartisan history of premium support. Walton J. Francis details the lessons from the Federal Employee Health Benefit

Program, which helped inform the creation of Medicare Advantage (chapter 11). Douglas Holtz-Eakin, PhD, concludes that reform based on premium support would result in both beneficiaries and taxpayers coming out ahead financially, while also allowing beneficiaries more consumer choice (chapter 12).

Medicare Advantage

The Platform for a Comprehensive Premium Support Program

Medicare Advantage (MA) is a health policy success. Created in 2003, this program is the alternative to enrollment in traditional Medicare. It is a system of competing private plans that provides comprehensive health care coverage, including catastrophic protection, and, in many areas of the country, delivers higher quality hospitalization and physician benefits and services at lower costs than traditional Medicare.

Since its inception, the program has experienced phenomenal growth. From 2003 to 2013, Medicare beneficiary enrollment in private health plans increased from 5.3 million to 14.8 million, or from 13 percent to 28 percent of total Medicare enrollment. Then from 2014 to 2021, Medicare Advantage enrollment grew 16.2 million to 27.5 million, or from 30 percent to 43 percent of Medicare's total enrollment. For 2023, the Medicare trustees estimate that almost 32 million beneficiaries will enroll in Medicare Advantage, accounting for approximately 48 percent of a total Medicare population of 66.6 million persons.[1] Over the past 20 years, then, this progressive expansion of private coverage and care has been steadily transforming America's largest health care payer.

The key to Medicare Advantage's superior performance is its defined contribution ("premium support") financing, whereby the government makes a per capita payment to competing health plans on behalf of Medicare beneficiaries. This superior financing is reinforced by the program's relatively flexible regulatory regime, enabling health plans greater leeway in the way they pay providers and administer health benefits.

These features distinguish Medicare Advantage from traditional Medicare. Traditional Medicare is a defined benefit system, where Washington policymakers determine benefits and medical services, and set prices and payments (both administratively and statutorily) through payment formulas, fee schedules, and price controls. Private health plans in Medicare must compete directly with each other in a consumer-driven market for the enrollment of senior and disabled citizens. They compete annually to provide traditional Medicare offerings and additional medical benefits based on quality, service, and premium price.

After nearly two decades of experience, Medicare Advantage has demonstrated superior performance in providing seniors high quality care at competitive prices.[2] Because of its superior record, Medicare Advantage has established a firm foundation for comprehensive modernization of the Medicare program based on consumer choice and market competition among health plans that is based on a system of defined contribution (premium support) financing.

Reform of the Medicare program, built upon the positive experience of the Medicare Advantage program, could attract widespread support among a broad range of health policy analysts, regardless of their partisan or political affiliation. Today, with the notable exception of "progressive" Democratic House and Senate members sponsoring legislation to outlaw private Medicare plans,[3] the Medicare Advantage program otherwise enjoys strong bipartisan support.

Building on Success

Congress can transform Medicare into a twenty-first-century health care program for current and future generations of seniors based on consumer choice, market competition, and defined contribution (premium support) financing. At the turn of the century, there was impressive bipartisan support for such a comprehensive reform, and that approach attracted majority support among the members of the statutorily created National Bipartisan Commission on the Future of Medicare, chaired by Sen. John Breaux (D-LA) and Rep. Bill Thomas (R-CA)

While the Medicare Advantage program has been a genuine public policy success, such a comprehensive transformation would require much more than a mere tweaking of the Medicare Advantage status quo. Medicare Advantage's record is one of positive achievements, particularly in the provision of broader benefit options and higher quality performance, yet it also highlights the need to eliminate some serious weaknesses. In pursuing Medicare reform, Congress should avoid replicating those deficiencies.

Specifically, Congress should:

- Fix the contribution system. Congress should replace Medicare Advantage's flawed and complicated system for health plan payment with a simpler defined contribution formula that would maximize health plan competition and beneficiary cash savings.
- Fix the risk adjustment system. Congress should remedy the deficiencies of Medicare Advantage's risk adjustment system, which still results in health plan gaming and plan overpayment—additional costs ultimately borne by beneficiaries and taxpayers.
- Broaden the competition. Congress should broaden health plan competition so that traditional Medicare, which accounts for almost two thirds of the entire Medicare population, competes with private health plans.
- Allow greater health plan flexibility. Congress should allow health plans greater flexibility in designing their benefit offerings and open up the competition to include new care delivery options.
- Block executive branch interference. Congress should erect statutory barriers to executive regulatory interference with consumer choice or health plan competition.

At the heart of America's continuing health care debate are differences over which approach can deliver the best outcomes for patients, as well as disagreements over the respective roles of government and the private sector. Interestingly, this division is manifest in the structural organization of Medicare itself. Whereas traditional Medicare is governed by government central planning and price controls, Medicare Advantage is powered by consumer choice and market competition.

The record is clear: choice and competition work.

How Medicare Advantage Works

Medicare beneficiaries can enroll in a Medicare Advantage health plan as an alternative to traditional Medicare. For *all* Medicare beneficiaries, there are a variety of private health plan choices. These include health maintenance organizations (HMOs), local preferred provider organizations (PPOs), regional PPOs (which are available to beneficiaries in any one of the Medicare Advantage program's 26 regions, including multistate regions), and private fee-for-service plans (FFS), where beneficiaries can choose any doctor who accepts the terms of the plan's contract.

Beneficiaries with specific needs, assuming they qualify under Medicare rules, can also choose certain specialized plans. These include special needs plans that offer benefits and services to persons—usually chronically ill, low-income seniors—with certain specialized health care needs. There also are "programs of all-inclusive care for the elderly" (referred to as PACE) for persons who require nursing home levels of care but who wish to remain in their homes.

Competitive Financing

Medicare Advantage's defined contribution system is its distinguishing feature. Under current law, Medicare makes a payment to health plans on behalf of Medicare enrollees. This payment program is a two-part process involving decisions by officials of private health insurers and the Medicare program.

First, the private health plans offer a bid set at an amount estimated to cover Medicare Part A (hospitalization) and Medicare Part B (physician and outpatient) medical benefits and services on a per capita basis. These health plan bids are proffered on the assumption that the amount would cover the costs of a beneficiary with an "average" health care status.[4] In different counties and regions with varying underlying resource costs, the costs of providing the traditional Medicare benefits likewise vary, and thus the health plans offer different bidding amounts in the various county or regional competitive areas.

Second, the Centers for Medicare and Medicaid Services (CMS) sets a benchmark payment amount for the Part A and Part B benefits for Medicare enrollees in their county of residence. The benchmark payment amount is to equal the maximum amount that Medicare can pay for Part A and Part B benefits. Under current law, this Medicare benchmark payment is further adjusted for the health risks that a health plan enrolls and the quality rating that the health plan achieves under Medicare's five-star rating system. The larger the number of higher risk enrollees and the higher the quality rating, the higher the Medicare benchmark payment for the health plan.

The Medicare program makes a per capita monthly payment to health insurers on behalf of their enrollees. The specific amount is determined by the relationship between the plan's bid and the Medicare benchmark at the county level.[5] If a health plan bids *above* the Medicare benchmark, then the plan can charge the enrollees additional premiums above benchmark to cover the additional costs that the plan would incur in covering the Part A and Part B benefits. If a health plan bids *below* the Medicare benchmark, then the plan must provide a rebate to the beneficiaries (between 50 percent and 70 percent) of the difference between the plan's bid and the Medicare benchmark; the remainder is remitted back to the Medicare program. By law the rebate must take the form of lower beneficiary premiums, reduced cost sharing, or the provision of additional health benefits.

Cost-Effective

Medicare Advantage plans generally offer traditional Medicare benefits (Parts A and B) at a lower cost than traditional Medicare.[6] In 2020, the Medicare Payment Advisory Commission estimated that Medicare Advantage plans on average bid at 88 percent of the cost of the traditional Medicare payments for Parts A and B benefits.[7] Research into the comparative performance of these Medicare programs also shows that Medicare Advantage's per capita health care spending ranges between 9 percent and 30 percent *less* than traditional Medicare, when it is adjusted for the mix of beneficiaries, including their health risks.[8]

Stable and Convenient

Medicare Advantage is a stable but dynamic program, with old plans exiting and new health plans entering, refreshing the pool of plan choices each year.[9] Like the popular and successful Federal Employees Health Benefits Program (FEHBP), Medicare Advantage is a thriving example of consumer-driven health insurance.[10] As Kristine Grow of America's Health Insurance Plans observes, "Medicare Advantage helps enrollees save money by capping out-of-pocket costs, offering additional benefits that traditional Medicare doesn't cover, and for many plans including comprehensive prescription drug coverage at no additional cost."[11]

Medicare Advantage also offers beneficiaries a simpler and convenient option for affordable, comprehensive, and integrated care, along with different cost-sharing and premium payments, including the option of paying no additional premium at all beyond the regular Part B premium payment.[12] In 2020, for example, almost two-thirds of all Medicare Advantage enrollees paid no premium other than the standard Part B Medicare premium required by the program.[13]

By contrast, traditional Medicare is structurally complex and confusing. With Medicare Part A, the hospital program, beneficiaries in

2022 faced an annual deductible ($1,556) and progressively larger out-of-pocket costs for hospitalization, and $194.50 daily for nursing home care following hospitalization. With Part B, which covers physicians' services, beneficiaries face a complex array of cost-sharing arrangements for many different services. Those enrolling in Part B must not only pay the monthly Part B premium ($170.01 plus a $233 annual Part B deductible) but also almost always choose to pay an additional private-sector premium for a supplemental or Medigap plan to secure crucial benefits not covered by traditional Medicare, notably catastrophic coverage. Beneficiaries may also pay a third monthly premium (an estimated average of $33.37 in 2022) for their Medicare Part D prescription drug coverage.[14]

Often Overlooked Savings

Following enactment of the Medicare Modernization Act in 2003, government actuaries and independent policy analysts complained that Medicare's payments to private plans were higher relative to Medicare's fee-for-service costs. Largely reflecting the impact of the payment changes enacted in the Affordable Care Act of 2010 (ACA), this payment disparity declined, and by 2017, Medicare's private plan payments equaled 100 percent of Medicare FFS costs.[15]

More importantly, Medicare Advantage delivers often-overlooked program savings, according to independent studies. The program's private health plans generate ancillary savings because they provide integrated and coordinated care and fill in crucial gaps in coverage that reduce overall program costs. For example, beneficiary enrollment in a comprehensive Medicare Advantage plan with catastrophic protection rather than traditional Medicare reduces their dependency on Medigap or other supplemental coverage to fill crucial gaps in coverage. A decreased dependence on Medigap would result in a decline in the excess utilization that today drives up overall premium costs in Medicare Part B and thus secure large savings to both beneficiaries and taxpayers.[16]

Medicare Advantage also helps offset Medicaid costs. A disproportionately larger number of low income and minority beneficiaries enroll in Medicare's private health plans, thus reducing their dependence on Medicaid and so reducing Medicaid costs as well. Black and Hispanic beneficiaries are contributing significantly to the growth in Medicare Advantage enrollment.[17]

Medicare Advantage's prevailing medical practice patterns also reduce overall Medicare costs. Specifically, managed care plans generate efficiencies that contribute to a reduction of costs in traditional Medicare.[18] This is the consequence of a Medicare Advantage "spillover" effect: physicians treating both managed care and traditional Medicare patients tend to adopt managed care practice patterns that influence their treatment of traditional Medicare patients.[19] Michael Chernew, professor of health policy at Harvard Medical School, and colleagues have estimated that a 1 percentage point increase in county-level Medicare HMO penetration was associated with an almost 1 percent reduction in "individual annual spending on fee-for service beneficiaries."[20] Though much more can and must be done to increase the economic efficiency of care delivery for America's seniors, the experience of Medicare Advantage, which is a working model of defined contribution financing, provides a strong basis to improve Medicare and secure future savings.

More Flexible Provider Payment

Medicare Advantage provider payment is also more rational because it better reflects market forces than the administrative payment formulas (including price controls) used in traditional Medicare. In traditional Medicare, government officials set and annually update over 10,000 prices for medical benefits and services in the Medicare program.[21] Because such administrative pricing cannot effectively reproduce the pricing of a free market, the Medicare payments for benefits, services, and medical devices are often set either too high or too low.[22] Moreover, this process of administrative pricing is further distorted by congressional micromanagement and intense special interest group lobbying.[23] In contrast, Medicare Advantage provider payments more accurately reflect real market conditions. As economists John Goodman and Lawrence Wedekind note, "Unlike ACO [accountable care organization] plans and traditional Medicare, where paying standard Medicare rates is mandatory, Medicare Advantage plans are free to pay higher rates to internists and other specialists to attract the services their patients need. Medicare Advantage plans can adjust to changes in market conditions; no other provider in Medicare can do that."[24]

An Eight-Step Plan Toward a Modernized Medicare Program

Congress can build on Medicare Advantage's successes. Washington policymakers can secure an even greater return on taxpayers' dollars, getting seniors better care for Medicare's heavy spending. To accomplish that objective, Congress will have to amend or repeal certain provisions of the Medicare law. Reform should make the Medicare Advantage program work better and enable it to become the foundation of a modern consumer-driven Medicare program for the twenty-first century that directly responds to patients' personal needs and preferences. Specifically, Congress must improve Medicare's financing and expand the range of beneficiary choices, while improving the program's cost control and ensuring an even higher performance in the delivery of quality care. To achieve these goals, policymakers should take the following eight steps.

1. Provide for Default Enrollment of New Beneficiaries into Medicare Advantage

Currently, any Social Security recipient eligible for Medicare Part A, the hospitalization program, is also automatically eligible for enrollment in Part B, the part of the program that pays for physician and outpatient services.[25] While Part B is a voluntary program, any eligible person receiving Social Security benefits is automatically enrolled in Part A and Part B, the traditional Medicare program. In short, under current law, enrollment in traditional Medicare is the default enrollment for persons eligible for Medicare coverage.

Based on the superior record of Medicare Advantage, particularly its provision of higher quality care for beneficiaries and potential fiscal benefits, Congress should switch Medicare's default enrollment for new beneficiaries from traditional Medicare to Medicare Advantage (as discussed in chapter 6). New Medicare beneficiaries could be automatically enrolled in the lowest cost, "premium-free" health plan in their county of residence, with the right to opt out of that plan and enroll in either Medicare Part B or another Medicare Advantage plan or some other approved private health plan.

2. Use Competitive Bids to Set the Government's Contribution to Beneficiaries' Health Plans

Congress should reform Medicare Advantage's defined contribution payment formula. It is both costly and unnecessarily complicated. Instead of basing the government contribution to health plans on the free play of cost-cutting competition among health plans themselves, the current formula ties the government payment to Medicare costs, which, in turn, are determined by the traditional Medicare's administrative price setting and controls for hospital, physician, and outpatient benefits and services. This arrangement is both economically and programmatically inefficient. As Urban Institute analysts have observed, "Evidence suggests that the Medicare Advantage benchmark and bidding system does not yield the lowest possible bids from insurers, which means the system is not promoting the most aggressive price competition."[26]

Congress should reform the existing defined contribution system by creating a new competitive bidding system that is simple and direct.

The new system should be based strictly and entirely on bids submitted by insurers for the amount they will charge to provide Medicare's benefits and services. The government's per capita contribution to insurers on behalf of Medicare beneficiaries—the "premium support"—would thus reflect the result of those competitive market bids.[27]

If implemented properly, such a new market-based bidding and defined contribution payment system would improve the efficiency and functioning of the Medicare program. The Congressional Budget Office, as well as independent analysts, find that such a program also has the potential to secure major savings for beneficiaries and taxpayers alike.[28]

Within a new competitive bidding system, there are several payment formulas that Congress could authorize to make premium support payments to competing health plans. While not exhaustive, there are three major possibilities.

First, Congress could pay health plans based on the average premium cost (or some percentage of the weighted average premium cost) of the competing health plans in a competitive area, whether that area is a county or region or some combination. This is roughly the same approach that Congress enacted for health plan payment for federal workers and retirees who are enrolled in the FEHBP; the government contribution equals 72 percent of the weighted average premiums of the competing health plans in the program.[29]

Second, Congress could instead authorize Medicare to pay competing health plans on the basis of the premium performance of the second-lowest cost plan in the competitive area. The Congressional Budget Office, among others, has already modeled this approach, and the use of the second-lowest cost plan would allow seniors to choose a health plan that is premium-free, just as they do today in the Medicare Advantage program.

Third, Congress could authorize Medicare to pay competing health plans on the basis of the weighted average of the three lowest-cost plans in the competitive area. This would also allow a choice of a premium-free plan.[30]

Before permanently switching to a new defined contribution (premium support) system, Congress should require CMS to undertake a demonstration program to test these three different formulas (and perhaps others) for establishing the best benchmark payment for competing health plans. Such a demonstration would enable policymakers to determine the best way to balance the goals of ensuring that health plans remain affordable for senior and disabled citizens, reduce the growing fiscal pressure on current and future taxpayers, and ensure market stability for the competing health insurance plans.[31]

Moreover, Congress should provide for a transition period, say, two or three years for the implementation of a new Medicare premium support program. During that transition period, Congress could prepare traditional Medicare to compete as a health plan and phase in the Medicare payment formula changes gradually, giving health plans, medical professionals, hospitals, and patients ample time to adjust to the new system and thus secure continued market stability and continuous coverage for Medicare beneficiaries.

Beyond testing different payment formulas, Congress should also require the CMS to determine the best geographical areas for competitive bidding among competing insurers. In the Federal Employees Health Benefits Program, the insurers pick their own competitive areas, reflecting where they have contracts with providers. Thus, it is not unusual for insurers to be operating in multiple counties or states. American health care delivery is undergoing rapid changes, especially with hospital consolidation, and care delivery is no longer confined to local or even state health care systems. Considering these rapid changes, CMS should determine whether to retain or expand upon the competitive county, multicounty, or regional areas for health insurance contracts, examining the continued usefulness of the 26 regions established in the Medicare Advantage program in 2003. Beyond traditional Medicare, which would remain a nationwide option for all beneficiaries, it may even be possible for Congress to create a new national market for private health plans, though it would require considerable work on the technical details, particularly regarding the allocation of health plan payment in different states and localities.

Three key principles should govern Congress as they create a new Medicare program based on defined contribution (premium support) financing:

- *Ensure that the government contribution is neutral in terms of the kind of plan a beneficiary chooses,* whether it is an HMO, a PPO, a private fee-for-service option, a health savings account plan, or a modernized Medicare FFS plan administered by the government. As the Medicare Payment Advisory Commission rightly prescribed, "The Commission maintains that to encourage beneficiaries to choose the model that they perceive as having the highest value in terms of cost and quality, the Medicare program should pay the same on behalf of each beneficiary making the choice. The Medicare program could not subsidize one choice more than another and still be financially neutral with respect to the beneficiary's choice to remain in the FFS system or enroll in a Medicare Advantage plan."[32]
- *Retain and improve upon the economic incentives in current law that encourage Medicare beneficiaries to choose the most efficient health care plans.* If a beneficiary chooses a plan that costs less than the government contribution, then the beneficiary pays no premium. If a beneficiary were to choose a plan that costs more than the government contribution, then the beneficiary would pay a premium to offset the difference. In each case, Medicare beneficiaries should retain the ability that they have today in Medicare Advantage to choose a premium-free health plan; the reformed approach would thus retain current powerful market incentives for beneficiaries to enroll in lower-cost health plans and thus exert downward pressure on program and taxpayer costs.

- *Retain an income adjustment for the government's defined contribution to health plans*, with progressively higher per capita payments for lower income beneficiaries. Under current Medicare law, beneficiary premiums for Medicare Part B, which covers physicians' services, and Medicare Part D, which provides drug coverage, are income related. Medicare Advantage is also financed by income-related Part B premiums. Upper income recipients pay higher premiums and lower income recipients secure larger government contributions to offset their premium and out-of-pocket costs.

Today, between roughly 4 percent and 5 percent of the total Medicare population, whether enrolled in traditional Medicare or MA, face higher Medicare premiums due to their higher incomes. Individuals and couples with annual incomes of $91,000 and $182,000, respectively, pay more than the standard rate of 25 percent of their total annual premium. Depending on the size of their income, high income beneficiaries would pay between 35 percent and 85 percent of the total annual Part B and D premiums.[33]

Conversely, lower-income Americans receive additional support. According to a 2022 report by the Congressional Research Service, certain categories of poor beneficiaries, about 20 percent of the total Medicare population, are eligible for government subsidies to offset their premium costs.[34] Most prominent are "dual eligible" enrollees: low-income persons with chronic illness who qualify for eligibility under both Medicare and Medicaid; for them Medicaid provides financial assistance for their Medicare or Medicare Advantage premiums, co-payments, and deductibles. Likewise, in the Medicare Part D drug program, persons can be eligible for a low-income subsidy that covers the costs of their drug plan premiums and cost sharing. In 2021, 13 million beneficiaries (27.1 percent of all Part D enrollees) qualified for this assistance.[35]

This wise and humane policy should be retained. For insurers, such income testing contributes to the stability of the market. For low-income beneficiaries, this adjustment ensures that health plan options remain accessible and affordable.

3. Replace the Medicare Advantage Rebate System with Cash Savings for Beneficiaries

One of current law's most attractive features is that it provides powerful incentives for beneficiaries to choose health plans that offer them the best value for their dollars. The empirical evidence is that they do just that. However, under current law, this economic incentive is confined to an unnecessarily complex and inefficient system of health plan rebates. Plans that bid below the Medicare Advantage payment benchmarks must offer rebates, a portion of which are earmarked for the Medicare program, with the remainder to be returned to the plans for distribution to the beneficiaries in the form of lower premiums or richer benefits. Under the ACA, the rebate system was modified to tie the size of the rebate to Medicare quality performance measures. Based on the Star Rating system, the largest rebates (70 percent) are awarded to plans that rank 4.5 stars or more and the lowest (50 percent) to plans with a rating of 3.5 stars. When bid below the Medicare benchmark (as most do), they must provide rebates that take the form of lower premiums or richer benefits for seniors. This unnecessarily increases Medicare spending.

This process should be simpler and more efficient. If Medicare beneficiaries choose health plans priced above the new competitively set government contribution, the beneficiaries should pay an additional premium to cover the additional costs, just as they do today. If beneficiaries choose plans priced below the benchmark, they should get a full rebate amounting to 100 percent of the difference between the premium price of the health plan and the new government contribution. Beneficiaries should be empowered to choose whether to take the difference in the form of a cash rebate or have the difference automatically deposited in a health savings account (HSA) that they would personally own and control, which would allow them to accumulate additional health care dollars tax free.

4. Fix Medicare's Risk Adjustment System

When a health plan enrolls a beneficiary, the plan agrees to cover the beneficiary's health costs. Those costs are determined by a variety of factors that contribute to higher risk. To account for these factors in adjusting health plan payments in the Medicare Advantage program, current law provides for a *prospective* risk adjustment system to determine risk before it is materialized in higher costs. Over the years, the Medicare Advantage program has improved its risk adjustment system; today's criteria for assessing risk includes the age, sex, institutional and Medicaid status of enrollees as well as their health conditions, including conditions diagnosed in the previous plan year. Enrollment of higher-risk Medicare patients in a health plan entails higher government payment to the plan.

While Medicare Advantage has improved its risk adjustment system over the years, Congress must require it to do better. After a series of audits, CMS found that some plans have been manipulating their risk scores for their Medicare patients, resulting in higher government payment. Such overpayments amounted to almost $30 billion over a three-year period.[36]

The central problem to address is the assessment and related cost impact of health risk. Medicare beneficiaries are older and sicker, of course, than the general population. Still, some Medicare beneficiaries are much sicker than others. Adverse selection occurs whenever a health plan enrolls a disproportionate number of higher risk ("sicker") beneficiaries with higher claims costs, such as a larger than anticipated number of chronically ill patients.

Unless the problem is properly addressed, the danger is that the disproportionately affected health plans must charge ever higher premiums to cover their higher costs, which in turn discourages the enrollment of additional beneficiaries in those plans, reducing choice and competition in the market. In the Medicare Advantage program, this process has not advanced so far as to threaten the Medicare Advantage market with the classic "death spiral" of health plans exiting the market and reducing beneficiary choice. However, it has resulted in very large and continuing overpayments in the program at extraordinary taxpayer expense.[37]

While Medicare Advantage has made genuine progress in this area, getting the "right" risk adjustment system for health insurance is a complex and difficult enterprise. Congress should create a *retrospective* risk adjustment mechanism for health status. This would be separate and apart from the other variables in the current *prospective* adjustment system. It is virtually impossible for Medicare plan sponsors or government officials to determine ahead of time which patients with poor health status—say, chronic conditions—are going to impose higher than average costs, and it does not logically follow that they will incur the same costs. As Edmund Haislmaier recommends in chapter 9, the best way to compensate for this problem is to add a retrospective mechanism—a risk transfer pool—that is designed to account for the cost and redistribute risk adjustment funds appropriately and equitably after the cost is incurred. Simply put, the payment system should be rooted in the hard data of actual claims experience.

A risk transfer pool would achieve the goal of market stability and allow for efficient cross subsidization of risks among competing plans and prevent "gaming" of the system. In such a system, all plans would be required to estimate the projected costs of persons with above average risks for enrollment in a common Medicare risk pool and then pay a negotiated premium to the pool to cover the estimated costs of these enrollees. Plan membership in the Medicare pool would be mandatory, but the pool itself, managed by plan officials rather than government officials, would be self-governing. Annual premium setting for the pool would be secured through deliberation and consensus among the health plans themselves. At the annual close of the enrollment year, any plan with a disproportionate enrollment of severely ill and high-cost patients would be made whole by the common pool.[38]

Improvement in the risk adjustment system would not only help beneficiaries with serious health risks gain access to affordable coverage, it would also ensure a level playing field for intense plan and provider competition that can control costs. Achieving these desirable goals is also facilitated by the defined contribution program itself. Medicare's premium subsidies for Part C and Part D are generous, each covering roughly three out of four dollars of total premium costs. This would enhance risk mitigation in a modernized Medicare program. There is also powerful empirical evidence from the FEHBP experience, which shows that the generosity of the defined contribution payment to health plans on behalf of federal workers and retirees tends to mitigate adverse selection, as does the broad flexibility that FEHBP plans have to manage risk.[39]

Regardless of the theoretical elegance of any risk adjustment formula, the true test is its workability. While policymakers must try and preserve good incentives for health plan participation, they must also avoid creating perverse incentives for plans to game the system and thus reward them for generating excessive costs at the expense of beneficiaries or taxpayers. Therefore, to minimize unintended consequences, policymakers should undertake a rigorous testing or demonstration of any new risk adjustment program before any systemwide implementation.

5. Broaden the Competition: Traditional Medicare Should Compete with Private Health Plans

Traditional Medicare today enrolls the vast majority of Medicare beneficiaries, yet it is still a 1960s-style system of fee-for-service payment, which inhibits its flexibility and its capacity to adapt to rapidly changing demands and circumstances. It is a complex set of disjointed and separately financed entitlements, its care delivery is fragmented, and its outdated administrative payment systems routinely reward medical professionals and hospitals for the volume of services rather than the value of those services. While beneficiaries must cope with a confusing array of cost-sharing arrangements, they are not even protected from the financial devastation of catastrophic illness. Such protection is the very point of having health insurance coverage in the first place.

Traditional Medicare should be modernized and compete directly with private health insurance.[40] In its current state, traditional Medicare, organized as a disjointed set of entitlements, cannot compete with integrated private health insurance plans. For the program to compete as a fee-for-service alternative to private health plans, Congress must transform traditional Medicare from a complex entitlement program into an integrated health plan. To achieve that goal, Congress should combine Medicare Parts A and B (the standard hospitalization and physician and outpatient benefits) into one program with one integrated benefits package, simplify its cost-sharing arrangements, provide catastrophic protection for Medicare beneficiaries, provide new managerial flexibility, and ensure the program competes directly on a level playing field with private health plans by financing it through the same defined contribution formula that is used to finance all other competing health plans.

Like private health plans, Medicare FFS would also submit a bid reflecting the cost of delivering the required package of benefits in the competitive area, and that bid would be included with others submitted by private plans in the bidding area for determining the government's defined contribution (premium support) payment to plans on behalf of the beneficiaries.

Congress should also test the market viability of recently established programs. For example, the accountable care organizations created under the Affordable Care Act should be required to compete on a level playing field with other health plans. Such competition would not only expand an informed and fully transparent consumer choice of these arrangements, but it would also improve the performance of ACOs.[41] Lanhee Chen of the Hoover Institution and James Capretta of the American Enterprise Institute observe, "These groups would compete directly with both Medicare Advantage plans and with the unmanaged traditional program. This would be a change from the current practice of assigning beneficiaries to an accountable care organization based on the affiliations of their primary care physicians, a process that leaves most beneficiaries unaware of the role accountable care organizations play in managing their care."[42]

Given different geographical market conditions and costs throughout the nation, traditional Medicare would, like private health plans, face both advantages and disadvantages in regional competition. America's health insurance markets are diverse, reflecting different conditions on the ground. In some parts of the country, traditional Medicare would secure a pricing advantage and in other parts of the country, private plans would dominate.

6. Allow New and Innovative Plans and Options to Compete

In a modernized and competitive Medicare program, Congress should also permit beneficiaries to choose new and different types of health care delivery options that meet Medicare's basic benefit and regulatory requirements. This would include not only employer-sponsored plans for retirees, which already participate in Medicare Advantage today,[43] but also health plans sponsored by unions and employee organizations and private associations as well as by fraternal and religious organizations and institutions.

Furthermore, Congress should allow for even more personalized medical care. Economist John Goodman, for example, suggests in chapter 5 that health insurers should be able to add a direct primary care component to their benefit offerings, which would enable seniors to secure same day appointments and day or night access to their doctors for a modest additional fee, if they wish to do so. Likewise, health insurers should be able to offer a self-directed care option for seniors who would like such a choice, where insurers could deposit funds into a patient-controlled medical account to cover personalized care or wellness programs.

Moreover, Congress should also allow beneficiaries to contribute to health savings accounts, which are often used in the employer-sponsored market. By 2022, these account assets exceeded $100 billion.[44] Unfortunately, Americans cannot continue to make these tax-free contributions to HSAs once they join Medicare—a silly restriction Congress should remove.

7. Allow Greater Flexibility in Health Plan Benefit Design

As noted, traditional Medicare has a set of defined benefits, and Medicare Advantage plans, as private plans, have the freedom to add other benefits, such as vision, dental, and various preventive medical benefits and services. In a modernized Medicare market, Congress would still require health plans to offer the standard Medicare Parts A, B, and D benefits as an integrated benefit package. It would extend to all plans a catastrophic coverage requirement, which is today solely a legal requirement for plans offering coverage in the Medicare Advantage program. Further, Congress should allow plans to offer different combinations of these benefits, as long as they provide the actuarial equivalent of this integrated benefit package.

There is already a working model for this kind of health benefit flexibility in the Federal Employee Health Benefits Program. Under current law, the FEHBP specifies the broad categories of health benefits that must be included in a health plan benefits package, such as hospitalization, physicians' services, ambulatory care, drugs, and medical devices. The detailed offerings, however, often differ widely from plan to plan. This is, of course, radically different than traditional Medicare's meticulously detailed requirements that govern its defined benefits, including thousands of medical treatments and procedures, and it would allow for far more flexibility in benefit design and care provision.

Today, Medicare Advantage already provides for specialized health plans, such as special needs plans, that enroll certain categories of patients with complex medical conditions or who suffer from chronic illnesses.[45] Patients in these kinds of plans get special benefits and are currently funded by separate payment streams. These plans should be continued for these special categories of patients, along with the financial arrangements that serve these patients.

8. Prevent Regulatory Interventions That Inhibit Choice, Competition, or Innovation

As a federal program, Medicare Advantage is governed by federal law and regulation, though the law and implementing rules are relatively flexible compared to traditional Medicare.[46] Under current law, health plans participating in Medicare Advantage must meet reasonable financial solvency requirements, demonstrate sufficient volume of enrollment, and comply with state licensure requirements.

In establishing a modernized Medicare program based on the Medicare Advantage experience, Congress should enact new provisions that would further protect the program's key competitive elements of consumer choice and market competition. These would serve as statutory guardrails against inappropriate, anticompetitive, or unwarranted presidential or agency interventions. There is a strong precedent for enacting such legislation. When enacting the Medicare Modernization Act of 2003, Congress included for Part D a preemptive statutory restriction on executive power—a noninterference provision—to protect private-sector negotiation between private health plans and drug manufacturers from executive branch interference.[47]

Similarly, Congress should extend that noninterference principle to the modernized Medicare program, based on premium support, and target those restrictions against government price controls, premium caps, or the imposition of federal government fee schedules on medical professionals in a modernized Medicare program. Congress should also prohibit the imposition of mandates of specific benefits, services, treatments, or procedures beyond the basic benefit requirements that are required for the process of competitive bidding. The provision of additional benefits should be solely determined by the competing health plans themselves in responding to patient wants and needs or the clinical recommendations of the medical profession.

Congress should also prohibit the administrative imposition of medical practice guidelines on doctors, hospitals, or medical professionals who contract with health plans other than the traditional Medicare plan; otherwise, all such medical standards for treatments and procedures should be left exclusively to medical professional organizations or be determined through independent contractual agreements between medical professionals and the competing health plans. The degree to which health plans wish to adopt government payment systems or practice guidelines should also be left to the plans themselves. For purposes of consumer information and engagement, such provisions in health plans should be fully transparent and thus subject, ultimately, to the judgment of Medicare beneficiaries as consumers.

Transitioning to a Modernized Program

In moving to a modernized Medicare program, Congress must address certain key issues, including the length of a program transition and the kind of governance that would be required for a new program.

Time Frame

Given that much of the infrastructure of a modernized Medicare program already exists, a transition period of two to three years seems reasonable. When Congress enacted the Medicare Modernization Act of 2003, it provided a three-year transition for the full-scale provision of a prescription drug benefit. Under the Affordable Care Act of 2010, insurers had four years to prepare for participation in the ACA exchanges that opened in 2014.

Enrollment

Congress must address the timing and eligibility of enrollment of Medicare beneficiaries. Current Medicare beneficiaries could be grandfathered in and permitted to remain in the current Medicare FFS program under current terms and conditions. Following the transition to a new modernized Medicare program based on premium support, those grandfathered beneficiaries should then be offered the option to enroll voluntarily into the new program. After the transition, of course, all newly enrolled Medicare beneficiaries would be free to enroll in any of the competing private health plans in the new modernized Medicare program, as well as an "enhanced" Medicare FFS plan (an updated version of the traditional program). The existing traditional Medicare FFS program, serving a diminishing cohort of older beneficiaries, would phase out with its steadily declining enrollment.

Competition and Governance

In a modernized Medicare system, all plans, without exception, should compete on a level playing field. For oversight of health plan competition, Congress should retain Medicare Advantage's governance structure. Today, the Center for Medicare, a subdivision of the greater CMS, administers the Medicare Advantage program, and the center gets administrative support from subgroups within the agency for data collection, enrollment, plan payment, oversight, and enforcement.

In this connection, it is crucial to separate the agency that administers the competitive market from the management of the government's Medicare FFS plan; an umpire should not be a player in the game. For the governance of the FFS plan, Congress should establish a board of directors, appointed by the president and confirmed by the Senate, that would manage and oversee the FFS Medicare plan, approve benefits, set premiums, enforce quality standards, and ensure consumer protection and information. The board should be given the managerial flexibility to enable the Medicare FFS plan to compete with private health plans in the new Medicare market.[48]

Looking Ahead

Medicare Advantage is a successful program. It is successful because it harnesses the free market forces of consumer choice and competition, enables patients to choose what they determine best for them, and delivers high quality care at affordable prices for Medicare beneficiaries. In structure and function, it is the opposite of traditional Medicare, an outdated defined-benefit system, governed by central planning and price controls, sluggish in response to change, and burdened with excessive bureaucracy, congressional micromanagement, and frenzied lobbying by powerful special interest groups.

Congress should build on Medicare Advantage's success and expand the defined contribution system to all of Medicare, thus creating a modernized Medicare program. In moving to such a premium support program, Congress can also remedy the deficiencies that today burden the Medicare Advantage program, such as a flawed government contribution and rebate arrangement and a flawed risk adjustment system. For Medicare beneficiaries, there are sound reasons to believe that these changes would result in a superior program.[49]

Such a reform would provide for a more granular level of patient choice and plan flexibility, thus allowing even more personalized medical services. Intense competition among a wider range of health plans and medical options would secure cost savings, revitalize employer-sponsored retirement coverage, stimulate innovation in both benefit design and care delivery, and encourage deeper patient engagement through more robust information and patient education.

Washington policymakers should not be deterred by comically outdated rhetoric that such a reform would "end Medicare as we know it" or amount to "privatization" of Medicare. Private health coverage is expanding rapidly already, and a modernized Medicare program, based on defined contribution financing, would be no less of a government program than Medicare Part C and Medicare Part D are today.

In the end, it is the patients that count. Current and future seniors can secure high value care in a modernized Medicare program powered by choice and competition, where the price and performance of health plans and providers are transparent, and information on both is readily and easily accessible for Medicare patients and patient advocates.

NOTES

1. Boards of Trustees of the Federal Hospital Insurance and the Supplementary Medical Insurance Trust Funds, *2022 Annual Report of the Boards of Trustees* (Washington, DC: Centers for Medicare and Medicaid Services, June 2, 2022), 157, table IV.C1, https://www.cms.gov/files/document/2022-medicare-trustees-report .pdf. Hereafter cited as *2022 Medicare Trustees Report*. See also, Meredith Freed, Anthony Damico, and Tricia Neuman, "A Dozen Facts about Medicare Advantage in 2020," Kaiser Family Foundation, January 13, 2021, figure 1, https://www.kff.org /medicare/issue-brief/a-dozen-facts-about-medicare-advantage-in-2020.

2. "Evidence from forty-eight studies showed that in most or all comparisons, Medicare Advantage was associated with more preventive care visits, fewer hospital admissions and emergency department visits, shorter hospital and skilled nursing facility lengths of stay, and lower health care spending. Medicare Advantage outperformed traditional Medicare in most studies comparing quality of care metrics" (Rajender Agarwal, John Connolly, Shweta Gupta, and Arnol S. Navathe, "Comparing Medicare Advantage and Traditional Medicare: A Systematic Review," *Health Affairs* 40, no. 6 (June 2021), 937, https://www.healthaffairs.org/doi/abs/10 .1377/hlthaff.2020.02149). While MA does not show a "trend of better performance" on such metrics as patient experience, hospital readmissions, or mortality, Agarwal et al. note that data quality limitations inhibit comparability in these areas and suggest that policymakers work to improve the data.

3. During the 116th Congress, Sen. Bernie Sanders (D-VT) and several leading Democratic Senators were sponsors of the Medicare for All Act of 2019 (S. 1129). A majority of House Democrats (118) sponsored the Medicare for All bill (H.R. 1384). For an analysis of the provisions of that House legislation, see Robert E. Moffit, "Total Control: The House Democrats' Single Payer Health Care Prescription," Backgrounder no. 3423 (Washington, DC: The Heritage Foundation, July 19, 2019, https://www.heritage.org/sites/default/files/2019-07/BG3423.pdf.

4. MedPAC, *March 2019 Report to Congress: Medicare Payment Policy* (Washington, DC: Medicare Payment Advisory Commission, 2019), 351, https://www .medpac.gov/document/march-2019-report-to-the-congress-medicare-payment -policy/.

5. MedPAC, *Medicare Advantage Program Payment System* (Washington, DC: Medicare Payment Advisory Commission, November 2021), 1, https://www .medpac.gov/wp-content/uploads/2021/11/medpac_payment_basics_21_ma _final_sec.pdf.

6. The Affordable Care Act of 2010 limits the allowable Medicare benchmark payment to MA plans in any given county to range between 95 percent and 115 percent of the countywide costs of traditional Medicare.

7. MedPAC, "The Medicare Advantage Program: Status Report," chapter 13 in *March 2020 Report to Congress: Medicare Payment Policy* (Washington, DC: Medicare Payment Advisory Commission, 2020), 367, https://www.medpac.gov/wp-content /uploads/import_data/scrape_files/docs/default-source/reports/mar20_medpac _ch13_sec.pdf. In 2021, the average MA plan bid was 87 percent of traditional

Medicare; see MedPAC, *A Data Book: Health Care Spending and the Medicare Program, July 2021* (Washington, DC: Medicare Payment Advisory Commission, 2021), 128, https://www.medpac.gov/wp-content/uploads/2021/10/July2021_MedPAC _DataBook_Sec9_SEC.pdf. Hereafter cited as MedPAC, *2021 Data Book*.

8. "Even at the lower bound 9 percent number, the savings are about three times larger than the most successful ACOs" (Vilsa Curto, Liran Einav, Amy Finkelstein, Jonathan Levin, and Jay Bhattacharya, "Health Spending and Utilization in Public and Private Medicare," NBER Working Paper no. 23090 (Cambridge, MA: National Bureau of Economic Research, January 2017), 86, https://www.nber.org/papers/w23090).

9. In 2016, for example, 87 percent of the plans in the MA market were also available in 2015 (Gretchen Jacobson, Anthony Damico, and Tricia Neuman, "What's In and What's Out? Medicare Advantage Market Entries and Exists for 2016," Kaiser Family Foundation, October 2015, 2–3, http://kff.org/medicare /issue-brief/whats-in-and-whats-out-medicare-advantage-market-entries-and -exits-for-2016).

10. For an overview of the success of defined contribution systems sponsored by the federal government, see Robert E. Moffit, "Expanding Choice through Defined Contributions: Overcoming a Non-Participatory Health Care Economy," *Journal of Law, Medicine, and Ethics* 40, no. 3 (October 2012): 558–73, https://www .employeebenefitadviser.com/news/hsa-assets-surpass-60-billion-growth -expected-to-continue. See also Jeet Guram and Robert E. Moffit, "The Medicare Advantage Success Story—Looking beyond the Cost Differences," *New England Journal of Medicine* 336, no. 13 (March 2012): 1177–79, https://app.dimensions.ai /details/publication/pub.1051766383; Walton Francis, *Putting Medicare Patients in Charge: Lessons from the FEHBP* (Washington, DC: American Enterprise Institute Press, 2009).

11. Quoted by Bruce Japsen, "Blue State Seniors Like Private Medicare Advantage despite Single Payer Push," *Forbes*, June 9, 2019, https://www.forbes .com/sites/brucejapsen/2019/06/09/blue-state-seniors-like-private-medicare -which-complicates-single-payer-push.

12. For an overview of the program's attractiveness to beneficiaries as well as insurers, see Robert E. Moffit, Rita E. Numerof, and Christen M. Buseman, "Let the Market Compete: Learning from Medicare Advantage to Move toward Value-Based Care," *Health Affairs Blog*, January 25, 2018, https://www.healthaffairs.org/do/10 .1377/hblog20180122.210298/full.

13. Freed, Damico, and Neuman, "A Dozen Facts about Medicare Advantage in 2020," figure 6.

14. All payments here cited are in 2022 US dollar amounts. See *2022 Medicare Trustees Report*, table V.E1 and table V.E2, 197–98.

15. Yash M. Patel and Stuart Guterman, "The Evolution of Private Plans in Medicare," The Commonwealth Fund, December 8, 2017, exhibit 4, https://www .commonwealthfund.org/publications/issue-briefs/2017/dec/evolution-private -plans-medicare. In this connection, it is worth noting that the Medicare trustees

project that the private plans' per capita bid trend is expected to continue to equal the average growth in traditional Medicare expenditures over the period 2021 through 2029 (see Boards of Trustees of the Federal Hospital Insurance and Federal Supplementary Medical Insurance Trust Funds, *2020 Annual Report of the Boards of Trustees* (Washington, DC: Centers for Medicare and Medicaid Services, April 22, 2020), 156, https://www.cms.gov/files/document/2020-medicare-trustees-report.pdf).

16. This is a widely shared observation among Medicare policy specialists. For the Heritage Foundation's analysis of the negative cost impact of current Medigap arrangements on seniors and taxpayers, see Robert E. Moffit and Drew Gonshorowski, "Double Coverage: How It Drives Up Medicare Costs for Patients and Taxpayers," Backgrounder no. 2805 (Washington, DC: The Heritage Foundation, June 4, 2013), http://thf_media.s3.amazonaws.com/2013/pdf/bg2805.pdf.

17. David J. Meyers, Vincent Mor, Momotazur Rahman, and Amal N. Trivedi, "Growth in Medicare Advantage Greatest among Black and Hispanic Enrollees," *Health Affairs* 40, no. 6 (June 2021): 945–50, https://doi.org/10.1377/hlthaff.2021.00118. See also Jill McKeon, "Medicare Advantage Associated with Better Minority Care Access," *PatientEngagementHIT*, August 17, 2021, https://patientengagementhit.com/news/medicare-advantage-associated-with-better-minority-care-access.

18. Michael Chernew, Philip DiCicca, and Robert Town, "Managed Care and Medical Expenditures of Medicare Beneficiaries," NBER Working Paper no. 13747 (Cambridge, MA: National Bureau of Economic Research, January 2008), 1, http://www.nber.org/papers/w13747.pdf.

19. Chernew, DiCicca, and Town, 2.

20. Chernew, DiCicca, and Town, 4.

21. Roger Feldman, Bryan Dowd, and Robert Coulam, "Medicare's Role in Determining Prices throughout the Health Care System" (working paper, Mercatus Center, George Mason Univeristy, Arlington, VA, October 8, 2015), http://dx.doi.org/10.2139/ssrn.3191400.

22. Federal agencies, including the Government Accountability Office and the Department of Health and Human Services's Office of Inspector General, cite many examples. According to the Congressional Research Service, "Numerous studies and investigations indicated that Medicare paid more for certain items of DME [durable medical equipment] and PO [prosthetics and orthotics] than some other health insurers and some retail outlets. Such overpayments were attributed, in part, to the fee schedule mechanism of payment" (Patricia Davis, Cliff Binder, Jim Hahn, Suzanne M. Kirchhoff, Paulette C. Morgan, Marco A. Villagrana, and Phoenix Voorhies, "Medicare Primer," CRS Report no. R40425 (Washington, DC: Congressional Research Service, updated May 21, 2020), 18, https://fas.org/sgp/crs/misc/R40425.pdf).

23. See Amitabh Chandra and Craig Garthwaite, "Economic Principles for Medicare Reform," *Annals of the American Academy of Political and Social Science* 686, no. 1 (November 6, 2019): 69, https://journals.sagepub.com/doi/full/10.1177/0002716219885582.

24. John C. Goodman and Lawrence J. Wedekind, "How the Trump Administration Is Reforming Medicare" *Health Affairs Blog,* May 3, 2019, https://www.healthaffairs.org/do/10.1377/hblog20190501.529581/full/.

25. Part B enrollment is allowable when eligible persons turn age 65, either three months before or after their birth date. Late enrollment is accompanied by a financial penalty equal to 10 percent of the annual Part B premium and is annually assessed as long as the beneficiary is enrolled in Part B. For a discussion on current options for seniors, see the Centers for Medicare and Medicaid Services, "Original Medicare (Part A and B) Eligibility and Enrollment," accessed July 8, 2020, https://www.cms.gov/Medicare/Eligibility-and-Enrollment/OrigMedicarePartA BEligEnrol.

26. John Holahan, Laura Skopec, Erik Wengle, and Linda J. Blumberg, "Why Does Medicare Advantage Work Better Than Marketplaces?," US Health Reform—Monitoring and Impact Report (Washington, DC: Urban Institute, January 28, 2018), 5, https://www.urban.org/research/publication/why-does-medicare-advantage-work-better-marketplaces.

27. There are different payment formulas for Congress to consider. The Federal Employees Health Benefits Program, for example, calculates the government contribution as a percentage of the weighted average of the premiums of all competing plans, with the "weighting" based on plan enrollment. Another prominent option is to base the government contribution on the second-lowest premium cost plan of all the health plans in the competition.

28. Different formulas would obviously yield different levels of savings for both beneficiaries and taxpayers. Beyond the use of an "average bid," for example, the Congressional Budget Office (CBO) also estimated the savings that would result from using the second-lowest cost health plan in a competitive area as the benchmark for health plan payment. This is also the plan payment formula for ACA premium subsidies in the health insurance exchanges. Examining both the "average" premium standard and the second-lowest cost payment scenario, the CBO reported that the range for just four years of savings (beginning in 2022) would be between $184 billion and $419 billion (*A Premium Support System for Medicare: Updated Analysis of Illustrative Options* (Washington, DC: Congressional Budget Office, October 2017), https://www.cbo.gov/publication/53077). Based on these CBO assumptions, Heritage Foundation analysts have estimated that the potential savings over the period 2020 to 2029 would range between $384.3 billion and $884.5 billion (*Blueprint for Balance: A Federal Budget for Fiscal Year 2020* (Washington, DC: The Heritage Foundation, 2019), 27, https://www.heritage.org/blueprint-balance). Such differences are why Congress should task CMS with conducting demonstrations to ensure the final payment formula achieves the best balance among the goals of lowering taxpayer costs, maximizing beneficiary affordability, and providing market stability for competing plans.

29. The Federal Employees Health Benefits Program has worked quite well and has been successful in keeping costs down and promoting choice for federal workers. Annual government contribution to health plans, as noted, is equal to

72 percent of the average weighted premiums of the competing health plans in the FEHBP market. For senior and disabled citizens in a new Medicare program, however, if such a percentage of the average premium were to be adopted as a payment benchmark, the percentage would be higher. It would reflect the current government subsidy for Medicare benefits, somewhere between 86 percent and 90 percent of the average of the competing health plan premium in any given year.

30. For further discussion of this payment level as an option for setting the defined contribution as the key component of Medicare reform, see Robert E. Moffit, "The Second Phase of Medicare Reform: Moving to a Premium Support Program," Backgrounder no. 2626 (Washington, DC: The Heritage Foundation, November 28, 2011), http://thf_media.s3.amazonaws.com/2011/pdf/bg2626.pdf.

31. Under the Medicare Modernization Act of 2003, the law that created the Medicare Advantage program, Congress authorized a demonstration program to test the viability of a new system of Medicare premium support. Unfortunately, the Affordable Care Act of 2010 repealed the provision authorizing that demonstration program.

32. MedPAC, *June 2014 Report to the Congress: Medicare and the Health Care Delivery System* (Washington, DC: Medicare Payment Advisory Commission, 2014), 5, https://www.medpac.gov/document/http-www-medpac-gov-docs-default -source-reports-jun14_entirereport-pdf.

33. Under 2022 law, upper income beneficiaries were projected to pay additional Part B monthly premiums in amounts ranging from $68.00 to $408.20; for Part D, their additional monthly premiums for drug coverage ranged from $12.40 to $77.90 (*2022 Medicare Trustees Report*, 199–202).

34. Patricia A. Davis, "Medicare Part B: Enrollment and Premium Costs," CRS Report no. R40082 (Washington, DC: Congressional Research Service, updated May 19, 2022), 24, https://crsreports.congress.gov/product/pdf/R/R40082.

35. "An Overview of the Medicare Part D Prescription Drug Benefit," Kaiser Family Foundation, October 13, 2021, https://www.kff.org/medicare/fact-sheet /an-overview-of-the-medicare-part-d-prescription-drug-benefit.

36. Fred Schulte and Lauren Weber, "Medicare Advantage Overbills Taxpayers by Billions a Year as Feds Struggle to Stop It," *Kaiser Health News*, July 16, 2019, https://www.stltoday.com/lifestyles/health-med-fit/medicare-advantage-overbills -taxpayers-by-billions-a-year-as-feds/article_433a8e61-7252-59b5-bd97-10437dc2 bec8.html

37. Schulte and Weber, "Medicare Advantage Overbills Taxpayers."

38. For a detailed description of this approach in creating a risk transfer pool for health insurance, see Edmund F. Haislmaier, "State Health Reform: A Brief Guide to Risk Adjustment in Consumer Driven Health Insurance Markets," Backgrounder no. 2166 (Washington, DC: The Heritage Foundation, August 1, 2008), http://thf_media.s3.amazonaws.com/2008/pdf/bg2166.pdf. Also see chapter 9 of this book.

39. On the FEHBP experience of dealing with adverse selection, see Curtis S. Florence and Kenneth E. Thorpe, "How Does the Employer Contribution for the

Federal Employees Health Benefits Program Influence Plan Selection?," *Health Affairs* 22, no. 2 (2003): 211–18, https://doi.org/10.1377/hlthaff.22.2.211.

40. In their *2014 Report to the Congress: Medicare and the Health Care Delivery System*, the Medicare Payment Advisory Commission observed, "The Commission has for many years supported giving Medicare beneficiaries a choice between traditional FFS and private plans under MA. The original goals for private plans in Medicare were to provide a mechanism for introducing innovation into the program while constraining Medicare spending. Private plans have greater flexibility to develop innovative approaches to care and can more readily use care management tools and techniques than FFS. If private plans reduce spending and improve the quality of health care services, then Medicare beneficiaries' ability to choose between the traditional FFS and MA plans can lead to great efficiency for the program" (5).

41. Avalere researchers note that in 2010 CBO projected that ACOs would secure an estimated $1.7 billion in savings between 2013 and 2016; in fact, the program not only failed to achieve such savings but instead increased federal spending over that period by $384 million. See Josh Seidman, John Feore, and Neil Rosacker, "Medicare Accountable Care Organizations Have Increased Federal Spending Contrary to Projections that They Would Produce Net Savings," Avalere Health, March 29, 2018, https://avalere.com/press-releases/medicare-accountable -care-organizations-have-increased-federal-spending-contrary-to-projections-that -they-would-produce-net-savings.

42. Lanhee Chen and James C. Capretta, "Medicare Reforms Both Parties Can Live With," *Politico,* September 12, 2018, https://www.politico.com/agenda/story /2018/09/12/medicare-reform-republicans-democrats-000695.

43. By 2021, 5 million beneficiaries secured coverage through employer-union group waiver plans, mostly managed care plans (see *2022 Medicare Trustees Report*, 156).

44. Greg Iacurci, "Consumers Have Saved More Than $100 Billion in Health Savings Accounts," *CNBC,* March 29, 2022, https://www.cnbc.com/2022/03/29 /consumers-have-saved-more-than-100-billion-in-health-savings-accounts.html.

45. For an account of the performance of these plans, see Jonathan Crowe, "How Competitive Private Plans Can Improve Care for Dual-Eligible Beneficiaries of Medicare and Medicaid," Backgrounder no. 2925 (Washington, DC: The Heritage Foundation, July 10, 2014), http://thf_media.s3.amazonaws.com/2014/pdf /BG2925.pdf.

46. As Dr. Scott Gottlieb, a former administrator of the Food and Drug Administration, has emphasized, "A combination of increasing regulation and declining reimbursement is leaving more and more providers reluctant to take on new Medicare patients. This, in turn, is leaving Medicare's fee-for-service program even more fragmented and making medical care harder to access and navigate for many seniors. The program's mounting regulation is also adding to paperwork requirements for patients" ("The Politics of Why Medicare Advantage Is Capturing Seniors," *Forbes,* January 23, 2015, http://www.forbes.com/sites/scottgottlieb /2015/01/23/who-benefits-as-medicare-burns).

47. This process of private-sector negotiation between competing health plans and drug manufacturers, a key feature of Medicare Part D, has been successful beyond expectations in slowing the cost growth of the Medicare prescription drug program. For a discussion of this precedent, see Senate Republican Policy Committee, "Medicare Part D: The Noninterference Clause," May 22, 2019, https://www.rpc.senate.gov/policy-papers/medicare-part-d-the-noninterference-clause.

48. Specifically, the board should be able to authorize new benefits and services, payment programs, and different combinations of benefits and cost-sharing arrangements that would enable the traditional Medicare plan to compete.

49. For a brief summary of the defined contribution patient experiences, particularly in FEHBP and Medicare Part D, see Robert E. Moffit and Alyene Senger, "Real Medicare Reform: Why Seniors Will Fare Better," Backgrounder no. 2800 (Washington, DC: The Heritage Foundation, May 20, 2013), http://thf_media.s3.amazonaws.com/2013/pdf/bg2800.pdf.

CHAPTER 8

Joseph R. Antos, PhD

Modernizing Traditional Medicare

The First Step to Effective Competition

Policymakers face a growing challenge with Medicare, the federal program that provides health coverage to nearly 67 million seniors and individuals with disabilities. Rapidly rising costs driven by perverse financial incentives and burdensome regulations have led to wasteful spending in Medicare that adversely affects the entire health sector.

Market-based reform can set the program on a more sustainable fiscal path and positively impact beneficiaries and American health care more broadly. The reason: Medicare is the largest purchaser of health services with leverage over the health system that will grow as the baby boom generation enrolls in the program. Efficiency-enhancing reforms in Medicare are likely to shape the professional and financial climate for the rest of the health care industry.

A comprehensive defined contribution system of financing—a "premium support" model—would align incentives in Medicare to promote efficient health care that better meets the needs of beneficiaries. That reform would replace traditional Medicare's uncapped entitlement and distorted fee-for-service structure with a uniform subsidy to purchase coverage from competing health plans. This would give all beneficiaries the opportunity to select lower-cost plans and give plans an incentive to provide necessary services in a more cost-effective manner.

For competition to work, all Medicare plans—including traditional Medicare—must be able to compete on equal terms. That calls for major reforms of the traditional program to better align with the offerings of Medicare Advantage plans. A critical first step is to simplify and modernize the traditional Medicare benefit, which does not meet current standards for comprehensive health coverage.

Unsustainable Spending and Perverse Incentives

Medicare's financial future is perilous. An aging population and the greater use of increasingly expensive—and effective—medical services will put unprecedented strain on the country's ability to finance the program. Medicare spending has outstripped growth in the economy over most of the program's history. Spending slowed following the 2007–09 recession but resurged in the past six years.[1] The Congressional Budget Office (CBO) projects that federal outlays for Medicare will double as a share of gross domestic product by 2050.[2]

That is optimistic. CBO's estimate assumes Congress will not override sharp cuts in payments to hospitals, physicians, and other providers scheduled under current law. The Affordable Care Act of 2010 (ACA) imposed a "productivity adjustment," which reduces Medicare payments to hospitals and other institutional providers by an amount that reflects productivity improvements in the general economy.[3] Those payment cuts cumulate over time, eventually endangering the financial stability of providers. Actuaries at the Centers for Medicare and Medicaid Services (CMS) estimate that by 2040 about 40 percent of hospitals, 66 percent of skilled nursing facilities, and 75 percent of home health agencies will be losing money each year as a result of the productivity adjustment.[4] These institutions and their medical professionals would likely cut back on the number of Medicare patients they serve as losses grow, despite any efforts they might make to reduce costs. The actuaries point out that "under such circumstances, lawmakers might feel substantial pressure to override the productivity adjustments."[5]

The Fundamental Problem

This impending crisis illustrates a fundamental problem with traditional Medicare. The program's uncapped entitlement and distorted fee-for-service structure are the major causes of the rapid rise in Medicare spending. Moreover, there is little meaningful competition among providers in traditional Medicare and little incentive for beneficiaries to seek out lower-cost care. As a result, there is little opportunity for market discipline to curb unnecessary spending or to promote efficient delivery of services.

Providers are paid for each of the services they deliver, giving them a strong incentive to deliver more, and more intensive (and more remunerative), services. Fees are set by the Medicare program, and participating providers accept those fees as payment in full. Nonparticipating physicians may charge Medicare patients 115 percent of the Medicare fee schedule (a practice known as balance billing), but most participate in the program. Price competition is essentially nonexistent in traditional Medicare.

Medicare beneficiaries are largely insulated from the cost of care. They are liable for deductibles and other cost-sharing requirements, which are intended to reduce program spending. However, over 80 percent of enrollees in traditional Medicare have supplemental coverage from private Medigap plans, employer retiree plans, or Medicaid.[6] Combined with Medicare's limits on balance billing, most Medicare fee-for-service enrollees pay only a small part of the cost of their care directly out of pocket.

Legislation to stem rising Medicare costs has focused primarily on lowering payment rates rather than changing the flawed payment mechanisms that promote excessive use of services. In fact, cutting payment rates may even exacerbate the spending problem if providers respond by prescribing more, or more intensive, services.[7]

The ACA promoted alternative payment models—including accountable care organizations (ACOs), value-based purchasing arrangements, and bundled payments for specific services—within traditional Medicare. Such strategies make providers financially liable for meeting government-prescribed performance measures intended to promote value over volume. Although these approaches can promote more efficient practice styles, they are simply layered on top of preexisting fee-for-service incentives and have had limited success in slowing the growth of program spending.

The results have been disappointing. The Medicare Shared Savings Program (MSSP), the largest of Medicare's ACO initiatives, resulted in higher program spending at first and only began to show savings in the last few years. In 2018, savings averaged $73 per participating beneficiary.[8] This is only 0.67 percent of Medicare's total benchmark spending per ACO beneficiary (approximately $10,900 annually). Bundled payment approaches implemented by CMS have had similarly poor financial performance. The bundled payment program for hip and knee replacements reduced spending by 1.6 percent from 2013 to 2016 but no savings have been found when bundled payment is used for other types of treatments.[9]

CMS has implemented more than 50 alternative payment models over the past decade, with only a handful of models generating net savings for Medicare.[10] Even the successful models can only chip away at the fee-for-service incentives that fuel traditional Medicare's spending growth.

Premium Support

The best alternative to the Medicare status quo is premium support—a market-based approach that replaces open-ended subsidies to beneficiaries and price-controlled reimbursements to providers with fixed-dollar subsidies. Beneficiaries could purchase the coverage they want from among competing health plans at the price they are willing to pay.

Under premium support, the business model would shift from one that is driven by volume and intensity of services to one that rewards cost-effective and efficient care.

Moving to premium support starts with a major reform of traditional Medicare. Although Medicare Advantage enrollment has increased rapidly in recent years, most beneficiaries are enrolled in the traditional program today and will be into the future. Over 36 million people were enrolled in traditional Medicare in 2021, and despite strong growth in Medicare Advantage, enrollment in traditional Medicare is projected to exceed 38 million by 2040.[11] Traditional Medicare is too big to ignore.

Reforming Traditional Medicare—and Medicare Advantage

Medicare is an amalgam of different kinds of health financing approaches that have not adapted well to the changing health care market. Traditional Medicare is a relic of the 1960s with only sporadic changes over the past 55 years to modify payment methods, update benefits, and make other changes short of a coherent reform. A more systematic approach would restructure the traditional program to bring the benefit up to modern insurance standards, promote efficiency and innovation in health care, and make the program fiscally sustainable for the future. Such reforms would enable traditional Medicare to compete fairly with Medicare Advantage plans.

Medicare is extremely popular with beneficiaries, despite its defects. Reforming, rather than eliminating, traditional Medicare is a practical first step toward a premium support system that offers beneficiaries a full range of health plan options. Such an approach addresses the dysfunction of traditional Medicare and changes the terms on which Medicare Advantage plans compete, creating new opportunities to reduce overall program costs while ensuring high value coverage for beneficiaries.

The following outlines major components of the first stage of market-based Medicare reform.

Modernize Medicare's Benefits

For a properly functioning health insurance market, consumers must be able to make an informed choice from the health plans that are available. That is nearly impossible for anyone trying to compare traditional Medicare's benefit with the benefits offered by competing Medicare Advantage plans. The traditional program's design is unlike any modern insurance plan, with complex provisions that provide inadequate financial protection to enrollees.

Enrollees in traditional Medicare face a confusing array of cost-sharing requirements that vary depending on the type of service. An enrollee requiring an inpatient hospital stay (covered under Part A) is liable for an initial payment of $1,556 (in 2022) for each "spell of illness" as well as substantial daily co-payments for extended stays. Some enrollees with multiple inpatient admissions could pay more than one hospital deductible in a year. In contrast, enrollees pay an annual deductible of $233 (in 2022) for physician and outpatient services under Part B and generally 20 percent of allowable costs above the deductible.

Adding to the complexity, enrollees are automatically covered by Part A, but Part B and Part D are optional benefits that charge monthly premiums (although nearly all beneficiaries enroll in Part B). Medicare Advantage plans cover all Part A and Part B benefits, and many also include coverage for outpatient prescription drugs. Unlike other health insurance (including Medicare Advantage), there is no catastrophic cap on out-of-pocket spending in traditional Medicare.

Cost sharing is supposed to make patients more sensitive to the cost of care. That does not work if the cost-sharing rules are incomprehensible, as they are today in traditional Medicare. A simpler benefit structure similar to most private insurance would be more understandable to consumers and would reduce the need for supplemental coverage to fill the gaps in Medicare coverage.

Several changes would be useful:

- *Combine Part A and Part B into a single program with a single premium that covers both parts.* Currently, the Part B premium pays for about 25 percent of the cost of Part B. Extending that to Part A would substantially increase program revenue, which would improve the program's fiscal outlook but substantially increase costs for beneficiaries. Lowering the premium to about 12 percent of combined Part A and Part B spending would be more affordable while maintaining the amount of premium revenue paid to Medicare.[12]

- *Simplify cost sharing and cap enrollees' out-of-pocket spending.* One possibility is to replace Medicare's current cost sharing with a single annual deductible of $700 for all Part A and Part B services, impose a uniform coinsurance rate of 20 percent for all spending above that deductible, and establish an annual out-of-pocket cap of $7,000. CBO estimates that this would reduce Medicare spending by $33.4 billion between 2024 and 2030.[13] To ensure that low-income seniors who do not qualify for Medicaid or other assistance are able to access necessary services, the out-of-pocket cap could be tied to income, with higher caps for those with larger incomes.[14]

- *Make prescription drug coverage a standard benefit* for traditional Medicare and Medicare Advantage, and cap beneficiaries' out-of-pocket drug costs as part of a broader reform of Part D.[15] Pharmaceuticals have become an essential tool in the treatment of disease, and drug coverage is commonly included in comprehensive health plans offered by most employers. Enrollees in traditional Medicare could continue to have a choice of competing stand-alone drug plans. Medicare Advantage plans would retain flexibility that they currently have in designing their drug formularies and other features of the benefit.

Reform Medigap and Other Supplemental Coverage

Supplemental coverage helps fill the gaps in traditional Medicare's benefits. Middle-class enrollees often purchase Medigap plans to avoid the uncertainty of Medicare's cost-sharing rules. There are 10 standard types of plans, with those offering more generous coverage charging higher premiums.[16] Two of the plans include an annual out-of-pocket limit but provide less complete coverage of cost-sharing requirements than the other types of Medigap plans.

By blunting consumers' sensitivity to cost, Medigap plans promote the use of services that could be obtained in less-costly settings, and that may not contribute to improving the patient's health. Moreover, Medicare as the primary insurer absorbs most of the cost of unnecessary services induced by Medigap coverage that reduces or eliminates what consumers pay out of pocket.

Congress could extend existing policy that prohibits Medigap plans from covering the Part B deductible for people who are new to Medicare.[17] One approach would prevent all Medigap policies from paying the first $700 of an enrollee's cost-sharing obligations for Part A and Part B services and limit coverage to 50 percent of the next $6,300 of an enrollee's cost sharing. CBO estimates that this would reduce Medicare spending by $59.7 billion between 2024 and 2030.[18] Combining this policy with the proposal to simplify Medicare's cost-sharing structure mentioned earlier would reduce program spending by $92.2 billion over that period.

Such a restriction could also be applied to supplemental plans offered by employers to their retired workers, but there are complications implementing this policy that are not present for Medigap policies. Benefits offered in an employer plan may have been collectively bargained and not easily adjusted. If those benefits offer the same coverage for retirees and active workers, a new federal requirement imposing a minimum deductible for retirees enrolled in Medicare would be difficult to implement.[19]

Another approach would be to require retiree supplement plans to operate as Medicare Advantage plans rather than providing wraparound coverage like Medigap plans. Such plans are known as employer group waiver plans (EGWPs), which exclusively enroll employer- or union-sponsored retirees and eligible spouses. They are paid a fixed amount by Medicare based on the bids of other Medicare Advantage plans available to individual (nongroup) enrollees.[20] Unlike Medicare Advantage plans, EGWPs do not submit bids and do not directly influence the capitated amount paid by Medicare. This reinforces EGWPs' incentive to seek lower prices and reduce the use of unnecessary services.

Promote Consumer Decision-Making

Consumers need better information to guide them in selecting their health plans, their doctors, and their courses of treatment. Steps have been taken to improve information on plan options and the cost of health services, but more needs to be done.

CMS offers online decision support tools to help consumers sort through their plan options, but that information is overly complicated and incomplete—reflecting complexity and gaps in the program. The Medicare Plan Finder makes it possible to compare premiums and coverage for stand-alone Part D plans, Medigap plans, and Medicare Advantage plans.[21] However, it is difficult to make a direct comparison of traditional Medicare (with or without Part D or Medigap) with Medicare Advantage. Information on retiree supplement plans is unavailable.

Most people new to Medicare are likely to get lost in the details, leaving them uncertain about the best selection to make from numerous options. How does one compare traditional Medicare, which requires separate deductibles for hospital and physician services, including the possibility of multiple hospital deductibles during the year depending on the patient's circumstances, with a Medicare Advantage plan that requires a single annual deductible? Would a Medigap plan be sufficient to fill in coverage gaps in traditional Medicare that do not exist in Medicare Advantage plans?

Reforming traditional Medicare's benefit structure would make comparisons with Medicare Advantage plans more transparent and give consumers a better idea whether a Medigap plan makes sense for them. Better information tools cannot overcome the confusion sown by traditional Medicare's complex and incomplete benefit design, but additional efforts to improve the information available to consumers could lead to better decisions.

Beyond the choice of plan, Medicare beneficiaries—and their physicians—need access to information about the price and quality of services on a real-time basis. Few patients shop for health care services like they shop for other products for two primary reasons. First, the health system is opaque. Patients do not have access to relevant information without having to laboriously contact providers and their insurer, and often the information they receive is incomplete or incorrect. Second, most patients rely on the advice of their physicians, who often have neither the information nor the incentive to refer the patient to a lower-cost, higher-quality provider. Moreover, physicians are unlikely to know which providers are in the patient's insurance network, they have no access to information about deductibles and coinsurance applicable to the patient, and most are not eager to discuss the cost of health care with patients.

This information dysfunction is endemic in the US health system and most acute in fee-for-service medicine. Two recent federal initiatives have begun to address this problem. The hospital price transparency rule, finalized in October 2019 and begun in January 2021, requires hospitals to post prices they charge various payers as well as a price list for "shoppable" services.[22] The transparency in coverage rule, finalized in October 2020 and slated to start in 2023, requires most health plans and health insurers to provide easy-to-understand personalized information on enrollee cost sharing for health care services as well as the rates they actually pay health care providers for specific services.[23]

Price transparency can promote effective competition that leads to downward pressure on prices in the private health care market. Price information can be used by employers to help workers shop for better value, particularly when the workers have a clear financial incentive to obtain care from lower-cost providers. The use of reference pricing, which sets a maximum contribution toward the cost of a medical service, has been effective in promoting price competition and shifting consumers to more cost-effective providers.[24]

However, requiring providers to reveal prices they have negotiated with insurers could exacerbate anticompetitive behavior in highly concentrated markets.[25] For example, knowing that competitors receive substantially higher payment rates from insurers could lead a lower-priced hospital to offer less favorable terms in subsequent negotiations.[26] Such actions can undermine selective contracting by insurers, which encourages providers to negotiate lower prices in exchange for increased market share. Whether price transparency leads to this perverse result depends on the extent to which insurers give in to the demand for higher payments, how much of the higher payments are transferred to consumers through higher out-of-pocket costs, and how price-sensitive consumers are to those costs.

These considerations are not relevant to traditional Medicare, which sets prices through regulation rather than through negotiation. Those prices are available to the public, but they are far from transparent to the average consumer. Medicare's fee schedules rely on detailed diagnostic and service codes that are difficult for someone without specialized knowledge to interpret accurately. Medicare's prices are not readily accessible in a user-friendly format, and medical judgment regarding the severity of a patient's condition is often needed to determine which of several payment codes may be applicable.

Even if the program's price information was more accessible and usable, that information would be unlikely to drive greater efficiency in traditional Medicare. Consumers are less concerned about the government's cost and more concerned about their own.[27]

As discussed earlier, out-of-pocket costs in traditional Medicare depend on complex cost-sharing rules and coverage limitations that vary depending on the service that is provided. They also depend on the type of supplemental coverage a beneficiary may have and the generosity of that coverage. Major reforms—modernizing traditional Medicare's benefit, restructuring Medigap plans, and improving information systems that more accurately estimate out-of-pocket costs—are needed to promote better understanding and better decisions by beneficiaries.

Making useful price information available to the public is perhaps the least difficult step toward promoting competition and value in health care. The more difficult challenge is finding ways to engage providers in helping their patients seek appropriate care in cost-effective settings. Heavy-handed regulation in a fee-for-service system is not the answer. Managed care plans, at least in concept, have an incentive to promote this sort of conversation, but success requires a cultural and financial change that aligns provider incentives with the interests of patients.

Improve Competition

As noted earlier, traditional Medicare is likely to remain the main source of coverage for large numbers of beneficiaries for the foreseeable future. Policymakers are unlikely to simply abolish that program in favor of Medicare Advantage, particularly since a key argument for Medicare Advantage is to let consumers enroll in a plan that best meets their personal needs. Even with its flaws, traditional Medicare is the choice of millions of Americans. Attempting to create a premium support system that abolishes traditional Medicare is almost certainly a political nonstarter.[28]

A strategy of benign neglect also makes no sense. Failing to enact reforms of the traditional program would keep traditional Medicare on an unsustainable spending path while exposing enrollees to inadequate coverage and declining value for money. Given that many people will continue to enroll in the traditional program, policymakers should take steps to reform what can be reformed.

More should be done to test new payment and delivery approaches in traditional Medicare. The lack of success for ACOs and bundling demonstration projects noted earlier reflects the top-down approach that CMS has taken. The CMS Innovation Center follows the federal procurement process that starts with the agency identifying the research project and specifying in detail the requirements for participating organizations. This limits the scope of innovation and restricts the organization's ability to adapt new ideas to changing conditions in diverse local markets.

To make traditional Medicare more responsive to changes in its own environment, the program should be open to greater entrepreneurship. Subdividing the program into regional Medicare fee-for-service plans, for example, would provide greater ability to develop and implement innovations that could reduce cost or improve value. Such regional plans could begin to operate as businesses capable of responding in a timely fashion to developments in local markets. High-level policy would continue to be set in Washington, but regional plan managers would have greater autonomy and be held to greater accountability for performance.[29] As currently structured, entrepreneurial innovation that responds to local conditions is the exception, not the rule.

Improving the operation of traditional Medicare would have an important and positive spillover effect on Medicare Advantage. The payment calculation for Medicare Advantage plans uses traditional Medicare spending as a benchmark, and that approach is likely to be retained under premium support.[30] A thorough reform would make traditional Medicare a more effective competitor, slowing spending growth relative to the baseline and lowering the Medicare Advantage benchmark payment. That would put additional pressure on Medicare Advantage plans to up their game.

Looking Ahead

Traditional Medicare's influence over the US health system should not be underestimated. The program's payment rules and regulations heavily influence how care is delivered to all patients, regardless of whether they are enrolled in Medicare. It is not surprising that traditional Medicare shapes the business of American health care. It is the largest single health insurance program in the country with nationwide coverage. Its policies affect nearly every provider, and they have the force of law.

New Medicare policies often respond to systemwide problems that should be addressed in a systematic fashion. The price transparency initiatives, for example, point in the direction of greater disclosure that is desperately needed. However, regulation can be a blunt tool where finesse is called for, and it is particularly difficult to fine-tune a regulation when there is a great deal at stake for providers, insurers, and consumers. Rather than relying only on the government's regulatory power, stronger market incentives are needed to ensure that reforms become part of the fabric of the health system. Reforming traditional Medicare is a good place to start.

• •

JOSEPH R. ANTOS is a Senior Fellow and the Wilson H. Taylor Scholar in Health Care and Retirement Policy at the American Enterprise Institute. He was formerly assistant director for health and human resources at the Congressional Budget Office.

NOTES

1. Anne B. Martin, Micah Hartman, David Lassman, and Aaron Catlin, "National Health Care Spending in 2019: Steady Growth for the Fourth Consecutive Year," *Health Affairs* 40, no. 1 (2020): 14–24, https://www.healthaffairs.org/doi/full/10.1377/hlthaff.2020.02022.

2. CBO, *The 2020 Long-Term Budget Outlook* (Washington, DC: Congressional Budget Office, September 21, 2020), 30–31, https://www.cbo.gov/publication/56516.

3. James C. Capretta and Joseph Antos, "An ACA Provision You've Never Heard of Could End Up Being Very Costly," *RealClear Health*, November 22, 2015, https://www.realclearhealth.com/articles/2015/11/23/an_aca_provision_youve_never_heard_of_could_end_up_being_very_costly_109431.html.

4. John D. Shatto and M. Kent Clemens, *Projected Medicare Expenditures under an Illustrative Scenario with Alternative Payment Updates to Medicare Providers* (Baltimore, MD: Centers for Medicare and Medicaid, Office of the Actuary, April 22, 2020), https://www.cms.gov/files/document/illustrative-alternative-scenario-2020.pdf.

5. Shatto and Clemens, *Projected Medicare Expenditures*, 7.

6. MedPAC, *July 2021 Data Book: Health Care Spending and the Medicare Program* (Washington, DC: Medicare Payment Advisory Commission, 2021), 27, chart 3-1, https://www.medpac.gov/wp-content/uploads/import_data/scrape_files/docs /default-source/data-book/july2021_medpac_databook_sec.pdf.

7. Christopher S. Brunt, "Medicare Part B Intensity and Volume Offset," *Health Economics* 24, no.8 (2015): 1009–26, https://onlinelibrary.wiley.com/doi/abs/10 .1002/hec.3081.

8. Jonathan Gonzalez-Smith, William K. Bleser, David Muhlestein, Robert Richards, Mark B. McClellan, and Robert S. Saunders, "Medicare ACO Results for 2018: More Downside Risk Adoption, More Savings, and All ACO Types Now Averaging Savings," *Health Affairs Blog*, October 25, 2019, https://www.healthaffairs .org/do/10.1377/hblog20191024.65681/full/.

9. Harris Meyer, "Bundles Cut Spending on Joint Replacements, but Not for Other Conditions," *Modern Healthcare*, January 6, 2020, https://www.modernhealthcare .com/payment/bundles-cut-spending-joint-replacements-not-other-conditions.

10. Chiquita Brooks-LaSure, Elizabeth Fowler, Meena Seshamani, and Daniel Tsai, "Innovation at the Centers for Medicare and Medicaid Services: A Vision for the Next 10 Years," *Health Affairs Blog*, August 12, 2021, https://www.healthaffairs .org/do/10.1377/hblog20210812.211558/full/.

11. Boards of Trustees of the Federal Hospital Insurance and the Supplementary Medical Insurance Trust Funds, *2022 Annual Report of the Boards of Trustees* (Washington, DC: Centers for Medicare and Medicaid Services, June 2, 2022), 181, https://www.cms.gov/files/document/2022-medicare-trustees-report.pdf.

12. Author's calculation based on *2020 Annual Report of the Boards of Trustees* (Washington, DC: Centers for Medicare and Medicaid Services, April 22, 2020), table II.B.1, https://www.cms.gov/files/document/2020-medicare-trustees-report .pdf. Note that the standard Part B premium is 25 percent of per-enrollee spending. Higher-income enrollees pay premiums that range from 35 percent to 85 percent of per-enrollee spending.

13. CBO, "Mandatory Spending—Option 17: Change the Cost-Sharing Rules for Medicare and Restrict Medigap Insurance," in *Options for Reducing the Deficit: 2021 to 2030* (Washington, DC: Congressional Budget Office, December 9, 2020), 25, https://www.cbo.gov/budget-options/56830.

14. Jonathan Gruber, "Proposal 3: Restructuring Cost Sharing and Supplemental Insurance for Medicare," in *15 Ways to Rethink the Federal Budget*, edited by Michael Greenstone, Max Harris, Karen Li, Adam Looney, and Jeremy Patashnik (Washington, DC: The Hamilton Project, Brookings Institution, February 26, 2013), https://www.brookings.edu/research/restructuring-cost-sharing-and -supplemental-insurance-for-medicare.

15. Several proposals have been advanced to simplify the benefit design for Part D and provide financial protection for enrollees. See, for example, Joseph Antos, Kirsten Axelson, and Sarah Rogers, "Medicare Part D Reforms: Who Wins and Who Loses?," American Enterprise Institute, December 15, 2020, https://www.aei.org /research-products/report/medicare-part-d-reforms-who-wins-and-who-loses/.

16. "How to Compare Medigap Policies," Medicare.gov, accessed October 1, 2021, https://www.medicare.gov/supplements-other-insurance/how-to-compare-medigap-policies.

17. "How to Compare Medigap Policies," Medicare.gov.

18. CBO, "Change the Cost-Sharing Rules."

19. Frank McArdle, Tricia Neuman, and Jennifer Huang, "Retiree Health Benefits at the Crossroads," Kaiser Family Foundation, April 14, 2014, https://www.kff.org/wp-content/uploads/2014/04/8576-retiree-health-benefits-at-the-crossroads.pdf.

20. MedPAC, *Medicare Advantage Program Payment System* (Washington, DC: Medicare Payment Advisory Commission, revised November 2021), https://www.medpac.gov/wp-content/uploads/2021/11/medpac_payment_basics_21_ma_final_sec.pdf.

21. CMS, "Medicare Plan Finder Gets an Upgrade for the First Time in a Decade," press release, August 27, 2019, https://www.cms.gov/newsroom/press-releases/medicare-plan-finder-gets-upgrade-first-time-decade.

22. CMS, "CY 2020 Hospital Outpatient Prospective Payment System (OPPS) Policy Changes: Hospital Price Transparency Requirements (CMS-1717-F2)," fact sheet, November 15, 2019, https://www.cms.gov/newsroom/fact-sheets/cy-2020-hospital-outpatient-prospective-payment-system-opps-policy-changes-hospital-price.

23. CMS, "Transparency in Coverage Final Rule Fact Sheet (CMS-9915-F)," October 29, 2020, https://www.cms.gov/newsroom/fact-sheets/transparency-coverage-final-rule-fact-sheet-cms-9915-f.

24. James C. Robinson, Timothy T. Brown, and Christopher Whaley, "Reference Pricing Changes The 'Choice Architecture' Of Health Care For Consumers," *Health Affairs* 36, no. 3 (2017): 524–530, https://www.healthaffairs.org/doi/full/10.1377/hlthaff.2016.1256. For a comprehensive review of research on how price transparency can be used to reduce the cost of employer-provided coverage, see Brian Blase, "Transparent Prices Will Help Consumers and Employers Reduce Health Spending," Galen Institute and Texas Public Policy Foundation, September 27, 2019, https://galen.org/assets/Blase_Transparency_Paper_092719.pdf.

25. Dionne Lomax and Sophia Sun, "Price Transparency: Friend or Foe? How Price Transparency May Impact Competition in the Health Care Industry," *Competition Policy International*, May 11, 2020, https://www.competitionpolicyinternational.com/price-transparency-friend-or-foe-how-price-transparency-may-impact-competition-in-the-health-care-industry.

26. Prime Healthcare has asked for a 14 percent rate increase from United-Healthcare for its New Jersey hospitals in recent negotiations, arguing that they have been paid rates substantially below the market. See Tara Bannow, "Coming to a Contract Negotiation Near You: Hospital Price Transparency Data," *Modern Healthcare*, September 23, 2021, https://www.modernhealthcare.com/finance/prime-unitedhealthcare-spat-shows-price-transparency-data-will-color-contract-talks.

27. Joseph Antos and Peter Cram, "Making Hospital Price Transparency Work for Health Care Consumers," *JAMA Health Forum*, April 5, 2021, https://jamanetwork.com/journals/jama-health-forum/fullarticle/2778428.

28. For more on the public choice dynamics of Medicare reform, see Mark V. Pauly's discussion in chapter 2.

29. Joseph R. Antos, Mark V. Pauly, and Gail R. Wilensky, "Bending the Cost Curve through Market-Based Incentives," *New England Journal of Medicine* 367, no. 10 (2012): 954–58, https://www.nejm.org/doi/full/10.1056/nejmsb1207996.

30. MedPAC, *Medicare Advantage Program Payment System.*

Medicare Risk Adjustment

Stabilizing the Market in a Premium Support Program

Medicare Advantage, Medicare's system of competing health plans, is the conceptual prototype for a Medicare program that fully leverages a premium support payment model. However, Medicare Advantage's current operational design was shaped by its origins as an offshoot of the traditional Medicare program. To fully transition Medicare to a premium support platform, policymakers will need to rework some of Medicare Advantage's operational components. In particular, policymakers will need to redesign the mechanisms used to ensure that plans do not have financial incentives to avoid enrolling sick people. Specifically, they will need to revise the payment formulas used to adjust plan payment amounts for cost differences among enrollees.

Currently, Medicare Advantage sets a base rate for payments to plans and then adjusts the amount to reflect enrollee risk. The base rate is set by looking at what is spent on beneficiaries in traditional Medicare (this is the "benchmark"); separate benchmark amounts and base rates are determined for each county where a plan intends to offer coverage.[1] The base rate amounts are then further "risk adjusted" using enrollee-specific data on health status and claims experience to derive plan payment amounts for each enrollee. This approach is intended to ensure that Medicare Advantage plan payments don't exceed county-level spending in traditional Medicare while also attempting to align payments with anticipated medical spending for each individual enrollee.

However, that approach encounters two sets of technical issues that policymakers will need to address in transitioning Medicare to full premium support. First, it will no longer be possible to use spending in traditional Medicare as the starting point for calculating plan payments. That is because under a full premium support model, traditional Medicare would be paid on the same basis as all other competing plans.

Rather than being a drawback, that it is actually an advantage of the premium support approach. Decades of government-administered price setting in traditional Medicare have produced innumerable, unjustified variations in provider payments and patient care. Premium support will give plans and providers the opportunity to start afresh without those distortions. It will also create an improved competitive landscape in which the plans that offer better cost and care outcomes can attract more customers. However, it also means that policymakers will need a different methodology for determining the base, or reference, value of Medicare benefits—in other words, the average value of Medicare's package of covered benefits before adjusting for any variations in plan designs and beneficiary characteristics.

The second technical issue is that the risk adjustment methodology currently used for Medicare Advantage has inherent, structural limitations that cannot be surmounted by simply doing more of the same or trying to do it better. Policymakers will instead need a different mechanism for adjusting for variations in medical spending among enrollees.

Over the years, Congress and the Centers for Medicare and Medicaid Services (CMS) have devoted considerable effort to trying to enhance the predictive accuracy of Medicare Advantage's risk adjustment methodology, but the results have been far from satisfactory. One big problem is that the current Medicare Advantage risk adjustment methodology tends to skew plan payments more to reflect the distribution of patients with chronic conditions than the occurrence of acute conditions. That is because chronic conditions—such as diabetes—are easier to identify in claims data or patient questionnaires, and the treatment costs of most chronic conditions are fairly predictable and constant over time. In contrast, the future occurrence of a major acute condition—such as cancer—cannot be predicted from past claims or health assessments. Furthermore, not only can the associated treatment costs be significant, but they can also vary widely over time. For instance, depending on the results of the initial treatments, the next year's costs for treating a cancer patient could be either significantly lower or significantly higher than those for the prior year.

The current system can result in delays to making payment adjustments up to a year or more after actual costs are incurred. This means that the current system can't effectively adjust plan payments prospectively for patients whose costs vary substantially from year-to-year.

While payment adjustments associated with these kinds of conditions will inevitably lag actual treatment costs, the current risk mitigation system is especially poorly equipped to address such situations. The current methodology relies on incorporating large volumes of enrollee-specific data on health status and treatment history. Not only are there wide variations in the predictive utility of the different data elements, but the collection and reporting of the data is also subject to errors, omissions, biases, and manipulations (both inadvertent and intentional) that can further diminish its value and distort resulting plan payments.[2]

To avoid those problems in a new Medicare premium support system, policymakers need to include payment methodologies and risk adjustment mechanisms that are based on fundamentally different approaches than the ones currently used for Medicare Advantage.

Objectives of Reformed Plan Payment and Risk Adjustment

Policymakers should design the mechanisms for setting and adjusting plan payments in a Medicare premium support system to meet the following objectives:

1. Ensure financial protection for beneficiaries, particularly those with expensive conditions.
2. Maximize the opportunities for beneficiaries to choose among competing insurers and different types of plans.
3. Incentivize insurers and providers to develop innovative plan designs and better approaches to care coordination and care management.
4. Enable insurers to offer plans that specialize in treating enrollees with certain conditions, such as cancer or diabetes.
5. Ensure that plans are incentivized to compete for enrollees not on the basis of health status but on price and quality, and to preference providers that offer better cost and quality outcomes.

Policymakers should also seek to minimize complexity and maximize flexibility so that the new methodology can better respond to a dynamic market characterized by continuous innovation in treatments and care. Policymakers should resist assuming that the path to success lies in gathering ever more data to use in fine-tuning the system to achieve ever more precise payment amounts. As past experience with both government payment setting in legacy Medicare and risk adjustment in Medicare Advantage shows, there are significant drawbacks to that approach. They include higher administrative costs, a greater propensity to generate inappropriate payment differentials that create financial incentives for undesirable behaviors, the unintended creation of opportunities for plans or providers to "game" the payment methodology, and structural rigidity that discourages or delays the adoption of new therapies and consistently lags in adjusting payments to account for increases or decreases in costs associated with innovations in medical treatments and patient care.

Structuring a Better Approach

The approach for setting and adjusting plan payments under Medicare premium support should consist of three sequential components:

1. A method for the government to quantify the base, or reference, value of Medicare benefits to serve as the starting point.
2. A formula for the government to then adjust the reference value amount into a set of per-beneficiary plan payment amounts that vary according to key predictive demographic characteristics.
3. A mechanism for the participating plans to adjust *among themselves* for the financial consequences of enrollee plan-selection decisions.

Step 1: Quantify the Value of Medicare Benefits

The first task is to create a new methodology for quantifying the base, or reference, value of Medicare benefits. That can be done by consolidating into one benefit package all of the benefits currently offered through Medicare Parts A, B, and D and then setting a minimum actuarial value standard—defined as the percentage of total average costs for covered benefits paid by the plan—for plans offering that coverage. For perspective, the most recent analysis on this topic indicates that Medicare's current actuarial value is about 80 percent.[3] In other words, of the total cost of benefits covered by Medicare Parts A, B, and D, Medicare currently pays on average about 80 percent, with beneficiaries responsible for the remaining 20 percent in the form of deductibles and co-pays.[4]

It will also be necessary to define the pool of beneficiaries used to determine actuarial value. The existing Medicare Advantage methodology operates at the county level, of which there are more than 3,000. In contrast, the methodology for Medicare Part D prescription drug plans is based on 34 regions, each consisting of one or more states.[5]

For premium support, the best approach would be to use the Part D regional divisions, or some variant thereof. First, each region encompasses a large and diverse pool of Medicare beneficiaries, thus ensuring statistically valid results when the data is used in the next step to adjust payment amounts to reflect beneficiary demographics. Second, regional divisions inherently capture geographic differences in basic economic factors, such as commercial rents and wage scales. Thus, determining reference value on a regional basis will automatically result in appropriate geographic adjustments that reflect legitimate differences in basic cost structure inputs common to all providers but will avoid reinforcing and perpetuating any unwarranted cost differences among competing providers in the same region.

The combination of a set of covered benefits, a minimum actuarial value standard, and a defined pool of beneficiaries will give insurance actuaries the basic parameters they need to design and price plan offerings.

Step 2: Adjust Payments for Demographic Differences among Beneficiaries

The second task is to construct a *simple* formula for adjusting each regional reference value amount into a set of per-enrollee plan payment amounts that reflect the key demographic characteristics that correlate with significant variations in average medical consumption. The most determinative of those characteristics are the enrollee's age and sex. In the case of Medicare, the next most determinative factors are the three categories of program eligibility (i.e., the aged, the nonelderly disabled, and those with end-stage renal disease) and institutional status (i.e., the institutionalized versus the noninstitutionalized beneficiaries).

There is a substantial body of data and analysis quantifying the differences in average medical consumption associated with these basic demographic characteristics. It therefore is a fairly straightforward process to construct an index for adjusting the reference amount to reflect the expected average annual costs of each group of beneficiaries with the same combination of demographic variables. Both the components of the index and the index as a whole can easily be updated on a periodic basis to reflect net changes in the cost of care over time. That is because the ongoing incorporation of new data into the dataset will automatically capture the financial effects of new treatments and care strategies, innovations in business practices, and changes in such broader factors as general inflation or the prices of key inputs, such as labor, rents, and utilities.

The result would be a simple table that lists for each combination of demographic characteristics the applicable ratio to be applied to the index amount in order to determine the plan payment for each enrollee based on his or her demographic characteristics. Policymakers should limit the prospective adjustment of plan payments to this set of basic demographic factors, all of which can easily be established and verified for each beneficiary. Beyond that, any further adjustments should be handled by the third component of the design.

Step 3: Enable Insurers to Adjust for Enrollee Selection Effects

The third component should be a mechanism that enables participating insurers to adjust *among themselves* for any skewed distribution of enrollees that might result from the plan selection decisions made by beneficiaries.

While the first component accounts for basic geographic variations and the second component accounts for broad demographic variations at the population-level, the purpose of the third component is to account for the aggregate effects of variations at the individual-level.

Even after adjusting plan payments to reflect demographic variations, uncertainty remains over which insurer and which plan each individual will pick when presented with a range of choices. It is possible that the collective effect of those individual decisions could be some insurers receiving a either a larger or smaller share of either better or worse risks—relative, that is, to the hypothetical result of each insurer's share consisting of a mix and distribution of risks identical to that found in the market as a whole. Addressing such uncertainty requires additional measures.

Risk Transfer Pool

Rather than attempting to predict and price the risk of each beneficiary, policymakers should adopt a "risk transfer pool" design that enables the participating insurers in each regional market to collectively adjust for any significant skewing among themselves in the distribution of risks and associated claims costs.

Risk transfer pools are preferrable to detailed prospective risk adjustment methodologies, such as the one currently used for Medicare Advantage, because they are less rigid and better support a market's ability to function smoothly. The key difference is that while prospective methods seek to engineer an *economic* outcome (alignment of plan payments with plan costs at the individual enrollee level), the retrospective risk transfer pool approach instead seeks to achieve an *actuarial* outcome: alignment of the distributional cost curve of each participating plan with the distributional cost curve of the market as a whole.[6]

For a Medicare full premium support approach, the market would be defined as all Medicare enrollees in a given region (including traditional Medicare enrollees as well as private plan enrollees). In each region, the risk transfer pool should do the following:

1. Apply to all insurers participating and all plans offered. Participation in the applicable pool should be one of the contractual terms that an insurer must comply with to offer Medicare premium support plans.
2. Be self-governing, with the participating insurers collectively establishing its rules and operations. While a pool might contract with third parties for administrative, accounting or analytic services, those entities would have no role in pool governance.

3. Stipulate that all participating insurers have equal rights (to cede risks) and responsibilities (to proportionately fund the pool).

4. Derive pool funding entirely from assessments on participating insurers (based on each insurer's share of the region's enrollees) with no external funding. The pool's purpose is to adjust among insurers for any significant skewing in the distribution of risks and costs—not to be a mechanism for obtaining additional, backdoor subsidies.

5. Operate under the regulatory supervision of state insurance commissioners.[7] Like medical providers, health insurers must be state licensed and regulated to participate in Medicare Advantage. That requirement should also apply to plans under premium support. Having state insurance departments oversee the risk transfer pools would further leverage the capabilities of state insurance departments (which already have experience with market-wide pooling arrangements in different lines of insurance). State supervision of the risk transfer pools would also ensure consistency with the other elements of insurer financial regulation.

The major benefit of this risk transfer pool approach is that it would force participating insurers—each with its own set of business considerations—to negotiate a mutually acceptable agreement on the details of the pool's operations. This approach leverages the reality that each participating insurer will inherently seek to avoid being disadvantaged relative to its competitors. No insurer will want to be uncompensated for attracting a larger than average share of high-cost enrollees. At the same time, each insurer will want to limit what it must pay in pool assessments by ensuring that the pool's design does not inadvertently undermine incentives for its competitors to control claims costs and improve care management.

Furthermore, because there is no single best way to design such a pool, an important additional benefit of this approach is that it encourages constructive innovations and variations that can be evaluated, adjusted, and organically evolve over time into a set of best practices. That is far more likely to result in an effective and smoothly functioning system than any attempt by federal Medicare officials to create and impose a single design of their own construct.

Looking Ahead

Such an approach to risk mitigation in a reformed Medicare program has the virtue of being simple, universally applicable, flexible, and self-correcting. It equips the private market to achieve what it does best: constantly innovate in treatments, care strategies, and business practices. And it does so through mechanisms that allow the market to smoothly and organically evolve over time.

• •

EDMUND F. HAISLMAIER is an expert in health care policy and markets at The Heritage Foundation.

NOTES

1. There is also a plan bidding process, and the base rate is set at the lower of either the plan's bid or the traditional Medicare-spending benchmark amount.

2. For examples of the inherent problems associated with the collection and manipulation of data inputs currently used to risk adjust Medicare Advantage plan payments, see US Department of Health and Human Services (HHS), Office of Inspector General, *Billions in Estimated Medicare Advantage Payments from Chart Reviews Raise Concerns* (Washington, DC: HHS, December 2019), https://oig.hhs .gov/oei/reports/oei-03-17-00470.pdf, and *Billions in Estimated Medicare Advantage Payments from Diagnoses Reported Only on Health Risk Assessments Raise Concerns* (Washington, DC: HHS, September 2020), https://oig.hhs.gov/oei/reports/OEI-03 -17-00471.pdf.

3. Frank McArdle, Ian Stark, Zachary Levinson, and Tricia Neuman, "How Does the Benefit Value of Medicare Compare to the Benefit Value of Typical Large Employer Plans? A 2012 Update," Kaiser Family Foundation, April 4, 2012, https://www.kff.org/wp-content/uploads/2013/01/7768-02.pdf.

4. Note that any Medicare premiums charged to beneficiaries, as well as any additional subsidies to help low-income enrollees pay cost-sharing amounts, should be addressed at the beneficiary level, not at the plan level. That way, Congress can ensure that beneficiaries receive appropriate financial assistance, while avoiding making the plan payment system unnecessarily complex.

5. The 34 regions encompass the 50 states and the District of Columbia. There are also five additional regions, one each for the territories of American Samoa, Guam, the Northern Mariana Islands, Puerto Rico, and the US Virgin Islands. See "2021 Medicare Part D Prescription Drug Plans: Overview by CMS Region," Q1Medicare.com, accessed December 4, 2021, https://q1medicare.com/PartD -2021MedicarePartDOverview-Region.php.

6. By transferring funds from plans that are "overweight" to those that are "underweight" at different places on the cost curve, the shape of the distributional curve can be made roughly the same for all plans and match that of the market as a whole. The effects of this risk transfer pool "norming" process would be to disincentivize competition based on risk selection (which shifts a plan's curve along the x-axis) and incentivize competition based on efficiency (which shifts a plan's entire curve down the y-axis).

7. As a practical matter, 25 of the 34 Part D regional markets consist of single states and each of the five territories also has its own insurance commissioner and is a separate Part D region. In cases where a region encompasses two or more states, the commissioners for the states in the region could agree to jointly supervise the pool. Alternatively, the pool could be domiciled in one of the states under the supervision of that state's commissioner. Either way, HHS would require insurers to participate in the applicable pool or pools where they offer Medicare premium support plans as a condition of participating in the program.

CHAPTER 10

Doug Badger

Modernizing Medicare

Improving Payment and Delivery of Prescription Drugs

Historically, a broad range of policy analysts and policymakers, both Democrats and Republicans, have proposed reforming the Medicare program through a system of defined contribution financing, commonly referred to as a "premium support."[1] In such a system, the government makes a per capita, income-related contribution to competing health plans on behalf of the beneficiaries, and the beneficiaries choose the health plans they determine best meet their personal needs. It is a model of consumer choice and market competition.

A Working Model

Medicare Part D, created in 2003, is the prototype of premium support. Medicare beneficiaries choose among competing prescription drug plans (PDPs): some freestanding, others integrated into Medicare Advantage coverage.[2] Drug formularies and premiums vary from plan to plan. The government subsidizes these premiums, providing low-income seniors with more premium assistance and better benefits. Beneficiaries with higher incomes receive smaller premium subsidies.

Premiums cover 25.5 percent of expected Part D spending for the year. Actual premiums vary from plan to plan, reflecting the difference between the plan's bid and the national average bid.[3] Seniors pay more to enroll in PDPs that submit higher bids and less to enroll in plans that bid lower. In 2022, the average basic beneficiary premium was $33.[4] The government computes its per capita subsidy payment to a PDP on the plan's bid relative to the national average bid, less the base beneficiary premium.[5]

PDPs prepare their bids based on the cost of providing a standard benefit to a beneficiary in average health. In 2022, the standard benefit included:[6]

- a $480 deductible,
- an "initial coverage limit" of $4,430,
- a "coverage gap" tier with up to $10,690 in total drug spending, and
- a "catastrophic" level, covering total drug spending above $10,690.[7]

The PDP must cover:

- 75% of drug expenses between the deductible and the initial coverage limit,
- 5% of drug expenses in the coverage gap, and
- 15% of drug expenses in the catastrophic tier.

The beneficiary is responsible for:

- 100% of costs below the deductible,
- 25% of spending between the deductible and the initial coverage limit,
- 25% of the costs between the initial coverage limit and the catastrophic tier, and
- 5% of the costs at the catastrophic level.

Drug manufacturers are required to discount the cost of their products in the coverage gap.[8] These discounts must offset 70 percent of a drug's cost in this range.

Manufacturers no longer offer these discounts once a beneficiary enters the catastrophic tier. The beneficiary pays 5 percent of the expenses in that tier, the PDP pays 15 percent, and the government covers 80 percent.[9] Thus, manufacturers and plans are responsible for only a small portion of the most expensive drugs' costs. This has created perverse incentives that are discussed at greater length below.

Private Negotiation

Drug prices are set through negotiations between PDPs and drug manufacturers. These negotiations are private and the arrangements complex, involving formulary placement as well as discounts, rebates, and other price concessions. Statute bars the government from "interfering" in these negotiations.[10] The government's role is limited to subsidizing prescription drug coverage for eligible beneficiaries. This "noninterference" provision has been controversial since the program's inception, with some arguing that the government could save money by directly negotiating prices with manufacturers.[11]

Government spending on Part D has been far lower than initially projected, suggesting that its reliance on private negotiations over drug prices is working. General revenue expenditures on the program in 2020 totaled $77.7 billion, less than it spent in 2016.[12] Over that same period, general revenue spending on Part B (physician and other outpatient benefits) grew by 41 percent (from $236 billion to $336 billion).[13]

The Part D program has also resulted in reduced spending elsewhere in the Medicare program by making drug therapies broadly accessible to seniors. Multiple studies have found that these therapies help keep beneficiaries out of hospital beds, physician offices, and emergency rooms, thereby reducing Medicare inpatient and outpatient spending. For example, the Congressional Budget Office (CBO) estimates that a

1 percent increase in prescriptions filled by Medicare beneficiaries reduces spending on medical services by 0.2 percent.[14] Applying the CBO methodology, Christopher Pope, PhD, of the Manhattan Institute estimated that an extra $100 in prescription drug utilization reduces Medicare spending on other medical services by $95 while delivering better outcomes.[15] Relying on different economic assumptions, economist Robert J. Shapiro in a 2016 study found that the Part D program had produced net Medicare savings of $679.3 billion between 2006 and 2014.[16]

While these estimates support the value of prescription drug coverage, most seniors had some form of coverage before the Part D program's inception. The comprehensiveness of this coverage varied. Some had retiree health benefits through former employers, which offered coverage comparable to Part D. Others purchased Medigap prescription drug coverage, which was not at all comprehensive. Others qualified for Medicaid, whose benefits varied widely from state to state.[17]

The Medicare Modernization Act (MMA), which established the Part D program, replaced Medicaid drug coverage for seniors with Medicare. Since the states and the federal government share the costs of Medicaid, the MMA required states to make annual "clawback" payments to the federal government to help fund Part D. In 2020, these payments totaled $11.6 billion.[18] The law barred Medigap plans from offering prescription drug coverage, beginning in 2006. To preserve employer-sponsored retiree drug coverage, the MMA established payments to employers. These payments, which were less than the cost of subsidizing Part D coverage, aimed to preserve employer-sponsored benefits.[19]

Medicare Part D's creation thus made prescription drug coverage voluntary, comprehensive, and virtually universal among the elderly.[20] To some extent, it also replaced other forms of coverage, like Medicaid and Medigap, and placed some of the costs of employer-sponsored retiree coverage on the government's ledger. Much of this new spending was offset by state clawback payments and reductions in Medicare outlays for inpatient and outpatient medical care, although estimates of these effects vary.

Perverse Incentives

Despite the program's relatively moderate spending growth rate and its offsetting benefits, spending in the catastrophic tier has accelerated. The Medicare Payment Advisory Committee (MedPAC), the agency that advises Congress on Medicare provider payments, estimates that gross spending (by beneficiaries, PDPs, and the federal government) for catastrophic benefits grew from just under $16 billion in 2010 to more than $68 billion in 2018.[21]

While drug plans, manufacturers, and beneficiaries finance prescription drug spending below the catastrophic tier, taxpayers shoulder 80 percent of the burden of the small minority of seniors whose annual drug spending falls into that tier (annual expenditures above $10,690).

That structure creates perverse incentives for manufacturers, plans, and beneficiaries with respect to the costliest medications. For example, PDPs bear 75 percent of the costs of prescriptions between the deductible ($480) and the initial coverage limit ($4,430), and so the incentive to make maximum use of their market tools—formularies, generic substitution, rebates, and price concessions—is strong in this tier.

Once a beneficiary's expenditures exceed this threshold, as it does for the most expensive products, that incentive weakens. PDPs pay only 5 percent of the coverage gap costs ($4,430–$10,690) and 15 percent in the catastrophic tier. They have little motivation to seek rebates and price concessions on the costliest medications.

Nor do manufacturers have much reason to grant them. They must provide a 70 percent discount on brand name products in the coverage gap, but once a beneficiary's spending rises to the catastrophic tier, they provide no discount at all. Thus, the higher a drug's price, the faster the beneficiary moves into the catastrophic level where no price concessions are required. This creates especially perverse incentives for drug manufacturers. As Tara O'Neill Hayes of the American Action Forum has noted in congressional testimony, "The mandatory discount decreases (as a proportion of a drug's price) as the price increases."[22]

MedPAC illustrated this point, using the example of the antiviral Harvoni, in its June 2020 report to Congress.[23] In 2018, the average gross spending per prescription for the antiviral was over $31,000, and Medicare Part D spent $1.7 billion in that year on Harvoni prescriptions. Total manufacturer discounts in the coverage gap for Harvoni amounted to just $17 million. That means that despite the 70 percent discount in the coverage gap, total discounts for Harvoni amounted to only 1 percent of Part D spending on the product in 2018.

The reason for this anomaly is that 89 percent of spending on Harvoni in 2018 occurred in the catastrophic tier. The federal government picked up 80 percent of this cost, plans paid 15 percent, and beneficiaries were responsible for 5 percent. Manufacturers have no obligations in the catastrophic tier.

An Emerging Consensus on Part D Reform

During the 116th Congress, a broad bipartisan consensus emerged around realigning incentives in the Part D program. While they differed from one another in detail, all of them sought to shift more of the burden in the catastrophic tier from the federal government to plans and manufacturers in the form of better incentives. This paper takes no position on specific proposals in these bills. Instead, it outlines a conceptual approach and offers some general policy considerations that lawmakers should weigh in recrafting the statute.

MedPAC's recommendations offer the contours of Part D restructuring. Specifically, its June 2020 report to Congress recommends changing the incentives placed in front of plans,[24] as follows:

- *Discontinuing brand manufacturer discounts below the catastrophic tier.* The 70 percent discount in the coverage gap has had the paradoxical effect of driving up spending at the catastrophic level. Manufacturers have responded to the statute's misaligned incentives by driving more spending into the catastrophic tier, where they no longer need to provide discounts. MedPAC recommends instead that plans cover 75 percent of the cost between the deductible and the catastrophic tier, with beneficiaries responsible for the remaining 25 percent. This would eliminate the "initial coverage limit" and create a seamless corridor below the catastrophic threshold.

- *Establishing a manufacturer discount in the catastrophic tier.* Requiring discounts in the highest tier would alter incentives for manufacturers. In contrast to the existing statutory arrangement, discounts would rise proportionately with prices. Consider the Harvoni example: MedPAC estimates that 89 percent of the $1.7 billion that Part D spent on that product in 2018 was in the catastrophic tier, where manufacturers provide no discounts. If the statute had required manufacturers to offer a 30 percent discount in that tier as MedPAC recommends, these discounts would have amounted to $454 million (27 percent of gross spending) instead of $17 million (1 percent of gross expenditures).[25] Of course, the manufacturer might have behaved differently if required to offer discounts that rise with prices. The purpose of the recommendation is to change that behavior by realigning incentives.

- *Increasing the plan's responsibility in the catastrophic tier.* Plans currently are responsible for 15 percent of a drug's cost at the catastrophic level and just 5 percent in the coverage gap. In addition to raising this to 75 percent between the initial coverage limit and the catastrophic tier, MedPAC recommends increasing the plan's share to 50 percent of catastrophic expenses. This recommendation, combined with moving manufacturer discounts into the catastrophic tier, would serve as a powerful motivator for plans and manufacturers to negotiate more reasonable prices for the most expensive products.

- *Reducing the federal government's share of catastrophic drug expenses.* The federal government currently bears 80 percent of the costs in the catastrophic tier, with plans and beneficiaries picking up the remaining 20 percent. MedPAC recommends reversing this dynamic by limiting the federal share to 20 percent and pushing 80 percent of the costs onto plans and manufacturers.

- *Establishing an out-of-pocket maximum in the Part D program.* Current law requires beneficiaries to bear 5 percent of costs in the catastrophic tier. There is no cap and thus no limit on what a beneficiary might have to spend in a year on prescription medicine. Elsewhere in this volume, we advocate for establishing an out-of-pocket maximum for Medicare Parts A and B spending, consistent with the role of insurance protecting against financial risk. Setting this threshold requires a complicated calculus. Currently, manufacturer discounts offered in the coverage gap count as "true" out-of-pocket spending. A restructured benefit would eliminate these discounts (along with the coverage gap itself). MedPAC and bills introduced in Congress suggest various out-of-pocket maximum amounts, generally falling in the range of $2,000–$3,000.[26]

Looking Ahead

This outline of Part D restructuring recommendations is conceptual and notional. Devising more specific recommendations is beyond this chapter's scope and requires a range of considerations. For example, legislation introduced on this subject to date generally required manufacturers to offer discounts both below and above the catastrophic threshold. Some tier these discounts to make them higher in the catastrophic level. Others require a uniform discount. Limiting the discount to the highest tier provides drugmakers clear incentives to hold spending below that tier. Requiring discounts at all levels would have an uncertain effect on these incentives.

The size of manufacturer discounts and the share that plans finance also require closer scrutiny. MedPAC estimates that had the 70 percent discount been in effect in 2018, manufacturers would have paid roughly $9 billion in annual price concessions.[27] One policy consideration would be whether to set aggregate discounts at comparable levels or to enlarge or reduce them.

Similarly, policymakers must consider the effect on premiums of requiring plans to bear a more significant share of Part D spending. While the restructuring described here would be of direct benefit to the small number of seniors whose expenses exceed the catastrophic threshold, this change might require all beneficiaries to pay higher premiums.[28] Better benefits (e.g., eliminating the coverage gap and establishing an out-of-pocket maximum) justify some increase in premiums.

In August 2022, Congress enacted the Inflation Reduction Act, which implements some of the reforms discussed in this chapter.[29] It caps annual out-of-pocket spending, beginning in 2025, at $2,000. It also reduces the government's share of costs in the catastrophic tier.

While these are positive developments, policymakers should closely examine these changes prior to their implementation. Specifically, the legislation elsewhere provides that the prices of certain drugs will be set by compulsory negotiations between manufacturers and the government, rather than between the manufacturer and prescription drug plans. This deviation from the premium support model will have an uncertain effect on prices for both generic and brand name drugs, as will the requirement that manufacturers rebate price increases that exceed the CPI-U, a measure of economy-wide inflation published by the Department of Labor. That requirement may serve more as a floor than a ceiling, particularly during periods of high economy-wide inflation.

Finally, the Congressional Budget Office (CBO) estimates that the Part D restructuring contained in the act would increase federal deficits by more than $25 billion over its first decade.[30] CBO estimated that legislation introduced in 2019 to restructure the Part D benefit would have the opposite fiscal effect, reducing deficits by $35 billion over ten years.[31] That is a troubling shift in the fiscal outlook for Part D restructuring and one that warrants the attention of policymakers.

Part D has functioned well by relying on competitive market forces to moderate prices and control overall spending, but as with any public or private program, it requires periodic review and modification. Recent changes to the program include some constructive reforms but also include modifications that substitute government negotiation for private negotiation in determining reimbursement rates. Policymakers should reconsider these changes and closely monitor their effect on prescription drug prices, access, and medical innovation.

Part D requires reform and restructuring that are consistent with its competitive market structure. Government price regulation is inimical to this structure. Choice and competition lie at the heart of its success. Reform should enhance these forces by realigning incentives.

• •

DOUG BADGER is a Senior Fellow in Domestic Policy Studies at the Heritage Foundation. He represented the White House in negotiations with Congress that resulted in enactment of the Medicare Modernization Act of 2003, which created Medicare Advantage and Part D.

NOTES

1. Henry Aaron and Robert Reischauer, both center-left policy analysts, advanced a premium support model in 1995 (Paul N. Van deWater, "Converting Medicare to Premium Support Would Likely Lead to Two-Tier Health Care System," Center for Budget and Policy Priorities, September 26, 2011, https://www.cbpp.org /sites/default/files/atoms/files/9-26-11health.pdf). The concept was embraced by a majority of members of the National Bipartisan Commission on the Future of Medicare. President Clinton appointed the commission, which was cochaired by then Sen. John Breaux (D-LA) and then Rep. Bill Thomas (R-CA). Because a supermajority of the commisssion did not vote in favor of the plan, the commission did not formally recommend it (Adriel Bettelheim, "The Last Time America Tried to Fix Medicare," Politico, September 12, 2018, https://www.politico.com/agenda/story /2018/09/12/medicare-bipartisan-commission-hoagland-lemieux-000693).

2. Medicare Advantage plans that integrate Part D coverage are known as MA-PD plans to distinguish them from freestanding PDPs. In both cases, participating entities submit bids for prescription drug coverage and meet other requirements, whether they are PDPs or MA-PDs. For that reason, throughout this paper we use PDP or simply "plans" to describe both integrated and stand-alone drug coverage products.

3. Centers for Medicare and Medicaid Services (CMS) first calculates a weighted nationwide average bid. The base premium is calculated at 25.5 percent of total expected Part D expenditures. The enrollee premium for a specific plan equals the plan's bid minus the nationwide average bid plus the base premium. Premiums thus vary based on the plan's bid relative to the nationwide average bid. See MedPAC, *Part D Payment System* (Washington, DC: Medicare Payment Advisory Committee, updated November 2021), https://www.medpac.gov/wp-content/uploads/2021/11/medpac_payment_basics_21_partd_final_sec.pdf.

4. CMS, "CMS Releases 2022 Premiums and Cost-Sharing Information for Medicare Advantage and Prescription Drug Plans," September 30, 2021, https://www.cms.gov/newsroom/press-releases/cms-releases-2022-premiums-and-cost-sharing-information-medicare-advantage-and-prescription-drug.

5. Government payments to plans are adjusted for several factors, some having to do with the characteristics of its enrollees. For example, the government will make larger payments to a plan that enrolls a low-income enrollee to cover the larger premium subsidy and the cost of providing more comprehensive coverage. Payments also are risk adjusted, providing larger payments on behalf of enrollees who are in poor health and can be expected to incur higher prescription drug costs. They also are adjusted for "reinsurance" payments, in which the government bears 80 percent of drug spending above a catastrophic threshold. Finally, there are risk corridor payments that adjust based on a plan's actual costs compared with estimated costs.

6. EBIA, "CMS Announces 2022 Medicare Part D Benefit Parameters Used for Creditable Coverage Disclosures," Thomson Reuters, January 28, 2021, https://tax.thomsonreuters.com/blog/cms-announces-2022-medicare-part-d-benefit-parameters-used-for-creditable-coverage-disclosures.

7. The $10,690 figure represents *total* drug costs, including those paid by the beneficiary and those paid by the PDP and the drug manufacturer. The actual amount a beneficiary spends out of his or her own pocket would vary based on that beneficiary's prescriptions.

8. 42 US Code 1395w-114a(g)(4). As originally enacted, the discount was 50 percent. Congress raised it to 70 percent for plan years beginning in 2019.

9. These are the percentages for brand name drugs. As discussed below, while PDPs are responsible for only 5% of brand name drug spending in the catastrophic tier, they must cover 75% of generic spending. This disparity contributes to the perverse incentives in the existing benefit structure, which make it in the interests of insurers and manufacturers to prefer high-priced drugs over more affordable alternatives.

10. 42 US Code 1395w-111(i).

11. During 2021, Congress was considering proposals to direct the Health and Human Services Secretary to negotiate the prices of certain drugs with manufacturers.

12. Boards of Trustees of the Federal Hospital Insurance and the Supplementary Medical Insurance Trust Funds, *2021 Annual Report of the Boards of Trustees* (Washington, DC: Centers for Medicare and Medicaid Services, August 31, 2021), 111, table III.D3, https://www.cms.gov/files/document/2021-medicare-trustees -report.pdf. Hereafter cited as *2021 Medicare Trustees Report*.

13. *2021 Medicare Trustees Report*, 91, table III.C4.

14. CBO, *Offsetting Effects of Prescription Drug Use on Medicare's Spending for Medical Services* (Washington, DC: Congressional Budget Office, November 2012), 1, https://www.cbo.gov/sites/default/files/112th-congress-2011-2012/reports /MedicalOffsets_One-col.pdf.

15. Chris Pope, "Issues 2020: Drug Spending Is Reducing Health Care Costs," Manhattan Institute, November 6, 2019, https://www.manhattan-institute.org /issues-2020-drug-prices-account-for-minimal-healthcare-spending.

16. Robert J. Shapiro, *The Value of the Medicare Part D Program for Its Beneficiaries and the Medicare System* (Washingont, DC: Progressive Policy Institute, December 2016), 5, https://www.progressivepolicy.org/wp-content/uploads/2016 /12/The-Value-of-the-Medicare-Part-D-Program.pdf.

17. Some states, for example, limited the number of prescriptions a recipient could fill in any month.

18. *2021 Medicare Trustees Report*, 111, table III.D3.

19. The MMA made these payments to employer-sponsored plans tax-free, thus increasing their value to employers. The Affordable Care Act, enacted in 2010, made them taxable. That change resulted in a sharp reduction in the number of employers who sponsored prescription drug coverage for their retirees.

20. Medicare Part D, like Part B, is voluntary. Some seniors do not participate, although many of them may have coverage from other sources, like a current or former employer.

21. MedPAC, *June 2020 Report to the Congress: Medicare and the Health Care Delivery System* (Washington, DC: Medicare Payment Advisory Committee, 2020), 128, fig. 5-3, https://www.medpac.gov/wp-content/uploads/import_data/scrape _files/docs/default-source/reports/jun20_reporttocongress_sec.pdf.

22. Tara O'Neill Hayes, "More Cures for More Patients: Overcoming Pharmaceutical Barriers," testimony before the House Ways and Means Subcommittee on Health, 116th Congress, American Action Forum, February 5, 2020, https://www .americanactionforum.org/testimony/more-cures-for-more-patients-overcoming -pharmaceutical-barriers.

23. MedPAC, *June 2020 Report to the Congress*, 130, table 5-1.

24. MedPAC, "Chapter 5: Realigning Incentives in Medicare Part D," in *June 2020 Report to the Congress*, 123–140. MedPAC also sets forth reforms to the

Part D low-income subsidy (LIS) program. The LIS is another source of Part D spending growth that deserves attention, but it is beyond the scope of my chapter.

25. This chapter advocates for a manufacturer discount in the catastrophic tier but does not endorse a specific percentage. The MedPAC example is intended to provide a quantitative illustration of how such a restructuring would better align incentives.

26. One design issue for policymakers to address would be whether to have separate caps on out-of-pocket spending for medical and prescription drug benefits or whether to create a single cap for combined medical and prescription drug spending.

27. MedPAC, *June 2020 Report to Congress*, 130. The discount in 2018 was 50 percent. Congress increased it to 70 percent beginning in 2019.

28. MedPAC estimates that 3.9 million people (8.3 percent of beneficiaries) exceeded that threshold in 2018. Of those, 1.1 million were non-LIS enrollees (MedPAC, *June 2020 Report to Congress*, 133, table 5-3).

29. "Inflation Reduction Act of 2022," H.R. 5376, August 16, 2022.

30. "Estimated Budgetary Effects of H.R. 5376, the Inflation Reduction Act," Congressional Budget Office, revised August 5, 2022.

31. "Preliminary Estimate of the Prescription Drug Pricing Reduction Act of 2019," Congressional Budget Office, July 24, 2019.

Reforming Medicare

Lessons from Premium Support's Long Bipartisan History

Federal health coverage programs have used premium support payment models since 1960 with the creation of the Federal Employees Health Benefits Program (FEHBP), now the largest employer-sponsored health insurance program in America with about 8 million enrollees. In 2003, after two decades of evolution, a largely mature version of premium support came to Medicare, the largest health insurance program in America with about 64 million enrollees and expenses that are now about 10 times larger than those of the FEHBP.[1] Forty-three percent of these Medicare enrollees are now in private Medicare Advantage plans, which (unlike traditional Medicare) are true insurance plans with explicit guarantees against catastrophic expense.[2] Understanding the history and experience of these two programs—each with successes and challenges—will help policymakers seeking to reform Medicare in order to lower costs and improve benefits.

Federal Workers' Coverage

The underlying model for premium support was first established by the Congress in the Federal Employees Health Benefits Program in

1960. The federal government as an employer was far behind large private corporations in providing health insurance as a fringe benefit. When the time came to remedy this problem, federal career civil servants and the Eisenhower administration copied the usual corporate model of the time in which one company (expected to be Blue Cross/Blue Shield) would provide health insurance in a "one size fits all" health plan.

But there was a hitch. Federal unions and employee organizations had already established or adopted a dozen or so health plans of assorted designs, including the Kaiser health maintenance organizations (HMOs), and they didn't want to lose their plans. In a classic case of one of the most fundamental rules of politics—the "grandfather rule," under which no constituency ever loses valued benefits already in place—the Congress rejected the proposed "one plan" scheme and devised instead a system under which the government would contribute a fixed amount (the "support") toward the premium of whichever plan each federal employee or retiree chose.

Thus, what is now called "premium support" was born. The insurance payer would allow many plans to compete for enrollment by employees. By paying a fixed amount somewhat less than an enrollment-weighted average premium, the payer would put an upper lid on its cost exposure and expect to save money over time by putting downward pressure on plan costs. While that fixed amount would rise to reflect higher costs for supplies and services covered by the insurance, it would be offset in part by cost-reducing management decisions. Each year each enrollee would either pay the difference between the fixed premium support amount and the premium cost of their chosen plan, or receive a lower price or rebate if choosing a lower-priced plan.

This is the way a market economy works, except that for most goods or services the individual customer pays the full cost. In the case of health insurance, employers or government programs pay most of the premium cost for enrollees. Using a premium support approach sets a ceiling on the subsidy and allows market forces to operate as if the enrollee was paying the full cost.

Medicare

Around the same time the FEHBP was created, another set of policymakers devised the Medicare program. Since the elderly then had no substantial or well-established set of existing insurance plans, political pressures did not oppose a "one size fits all" approach; traditional Medicare was enacted with a single plan administered by the federal government itself rather than a private insurance company acting as a manager on behalf of the government (private companies were used, however, as clerical bill payers).

This original Medicare plan had two semi-independent parts following the custom of the times (long since abandoned by every other health insurance plan in America), and thus "Part A" for hospital payments and "Part B" for physician and related medical service payments were created. They remain separate to this day with different payment rules, different financing arrangements, and different cost-sharing requirements for enrollees to meet. Moreover, Medicare is not actually an insurance program, as that term is otherwise universally understood, because it sets no upper limit on costs that enrollees may have to pay, and thereby fails the most important purpose of insurance: to prevent financial catastrophe.[3]

So defective is Medicare's design as an insurance program that 48 percent of its enrollees now choose private health plans that offer true insurance under the Medicare Advantage program (as created in 2003 and evolved since then), a program administered via a form of premium support. Ninety percent of the rest obtain substantial financial protection from either Medigap plans, employer supplementation plans that operate similarly to Medigap plans, or simultaneous enrollment in Medicaid and Medicare for those who are dual eligible.

Medicare Advantage

The Medicare Modernization Act of 2003 partially addressed the problems of traditional Medicare by creating Medicare Advantage and

Part D (drug coverage) and using a form of premium support to expand the role of private plans as competitors to traditional Medicare, while adding drug benefits and maximum out-of-pocket limit protection to the menu of offerings (initially for some of these plans and a few years later for all). Very importantly for competition among private plans, it created an "open season" enrollment period in which plans would compete for enrollees and enrollees commit to at least a one-year enrollment in the plan they selected (under the predecessor program enrollees could and would switch health plans during the year). Finally, the competition incentives were soon modified to reward enrollees in lower-cost plans with premium reductions or supplemental benefits.

These changes were not a complete break with the past, since private plan participation in Medicare had been evolving over time, but these features taken together were a revolutionary change. In particular, for the first time since Medicare was created, all Medicare beneficiaries could now enroll in essentially free "zero premium" insurance plan options that protected them from financial risk, without paying for expensive Medigap insurance as a substantial but incomplete protection. As I'll discuss later in this chapter, it also created a major cost reduction reform for traditional Medicare by eliminating the massive overutilization of medical care by enrollees who had first-dollar coverage from Medigap and former employer plans.

Support for Leveraging Premium Support Models for Broader Medicare Reform

Liberal and conservative experts and elected policymakers have long proposed using a broader form of premium support in Medicare (beyond that used today) to slow the rate of cost growth in Medicare while maintaining or improving medical care.

Academic Experts

In 1995, *Health Affairs* devoted an issue to this topic and several different authors, including Henry Aaron and Robert Reischauer from the liberal side and Stuart Butler and Robert Moffit from the conservative side, proposed reforms with similar contours for Medicare reform.[4] In 1999, former Medicare administrator Gail Wilensky and Harvard University professor Joseph Newhouse presented a variation of premium support, laying out the dimensions of design and arguing that age-rating of premiums would allow expansion of Medicare to a younger eligibility age.[5] In 2008, University of Pennsylvania economist Mark Pauly, in *Markets Without Magic: How Competition Might Save Medicare*, laid out in detail how a competitive system of plan bids with traditional Medicare as another plan could work, drawing on the early successes of Medicare Advantage and Medicare Part D.[6] A year later, a trio of economists published *Bring Market Prices to Medicare*, with an even more detailed set of recommendations focused on plan bids and plan competition.[7] In 2011, Alice Rivlin of the Brookings Institution and former Senator Pete Domenici of New Mexico published a proposal under the Bipartisan Policy Center.[8]

Elected Policymakers

Bipartisan support occurred in Congress, too. In 1999, for example, the National Bipartisan Commission on the Future of Medicare (widely known as the Breaux-Thomas Commission) came within one vote of agreement. In 2011, Sen. Ron Wyden (D-OR) and Rep. Paul Ryan (R-WI), two expert Congressional proponents of strengthening Medicare, proposed a premium support system, with special attention to features protecting enrollees from benefit cutbacks or excessive premium increases.

How Premium Support Works

How then does this premium support model work in the FEHBP and Medicare Advantage? Under the FEHBP, a substantial number of insurance plans compete to attract enrollment from government employees and retirees. Each employee is given a wide choice of plans and is responsible for choosing the plan that best meets his or her needs and budget. Plans must meet broad coverage standards but can fine-tune benefit choices, cost sharing, network, and plan red tape for handling bills and getting approval for some services.[9] More expensive benefits require higher premiums, unless offset by cost-reducing measures. Plan decisions are tested by how attractive each plan's mix is in attracting enrollees while in competition with other plans. A one-month open season each fall allows each enrollee the option of changing to any other plan serving his area for the coming year, with no preexisting condition exclusions.

The government sets a ceiling support amount for different family sizes and pays up to that amount toward the premium cost of any of these health insurance plans in the FEHBP. That amount is set as a fraction of the enrollment-weighted average premium of all participating plans. The resulting "support" level is identical no matter which plan enrolls any particular employee or family, varying only by simple actuarial risk factors, namely whether the enrollment is for self only, self plus one person, or a family of two or more. Any premium cost above that set amount in the particular plan a person (or family) enrolls in is paid by the enrollee. If the enrollee chooses a plan whose premium is below that support amount, the enrollee's premium is reduced by some fraction of the resulting saving. This means enrollees pay the full marginal cost of their insurance plan choices, which creates incentives for plans to control costs, bring premiums down, and improve benefits—and in striving for these goals, to become better buys and be more successful in attracting enrollees.

With Medicare Advantage, premium support occurs in a partial way. A premium support level is set by averaging the premium bids from participating private plans. Medicare enrollees can choose one of these plans in an annual open season. If enrollees choose a plan below the premium support amount, they receive either lower health plan premiums (often in the form of paying the Part D drug benefit premium), expanded benefits, or both.

These program designs are in large part (though with some large defects) the way private markets work normally. The designs have major effects not only on costs but also on customer satisfaction with the benefits and services provided. For example, in a competitive market, health plans have a strong incentive to provide economical generic drugs at a lower cost to enrollees than brand drugs, and both enrollees and the plan benefit from those lower cost choices. The details of those choices are made by plans, not by government bureaucrats or Congress, and modified each year by plans responding to consumer choices.

Imperfect Competition: The FEHBP and Medicare Advantage as Models for Premium Support

How well do the FEHBP and Medicare Advantage meet the ideal premium support model? Imperfectly. The areas where they fall short offer policymakers ripe ground to introduce reforms that build on and extend the programs' successes.

Medicare Advantage Defects

The biggest areas of imperfect competition with regards to Medicare Advantage (MA) are the presence of Medigap plans and similar "wraparound" employer plans for their retirees, which badly distort incentives for both enrollees and plans by raising the cost of traditional Medicare through excess utilization of unnecessary medical care. This in turn provides a cushion of bloat that protects MA plans from the competition that a "leaner and meaner" Medicare program could supply.

Another major defect is that traditional Medicare distorts the competition between that program and Medicare Advantage plans, leading to incomplete research findings that MA plans cost rather than save money compared to traditional Medicare. Medicare's failure to include true insurance against financially disastrous health care costs is a major factor that leads many enrollees to Medigap plans and many generous former employers to offer wraparound plans to their retirees. Because Medicare is "primary," the supplemental protection (from either Medigap or retirement plans from prior employers) increases Medicare costs by reducing or eliminating cost sharing and reducing or eliminating enrollee incentives to consider relative costs between providers or treatments as a decision factor in health choices. But by enabling enrollees to avoid Medigap plans, Medicare Advantage plans not only offer substantial premium savings to enrollees but also generate savings to traditional Medicare of several thousand dollars a year per enrollee (see further analysis later in this chapter). However desirable this makes Medicare Advantage on budgetary grounds, it prevents an apples-to-apples comparison among Medicare and Medicare Advantage plan choices by enrollees.

FEHBP Defects

The major defects of the FEHBP start with it suffering badly due to the lack of risk adjustment to level the playing field between plans with higher or lower proportions of more or less expensive enrollees.[10] The effects of this defect are magnified substantially because employees and retirees are in the same risk pool, with no adjustment being made for either age or enrollment in Medicare. What this means in practice is that plans that do an exceptional job in keeping their costs low, such as the Kaiser HMO plans, attract a disproportionate number of aged retirees who forgo Medicare Part B. This forces these plans to raise premiums to cover costs that Medicare would pay, thereby reducing the attractiveness of their plans to young and healthy employees. Most FEHBP plans also provide a wraparound feature that operates essentially the same as Medigap plans, eliminating cost reduction incentives for enrollees while raising costs to Medicare, the primary payer.

Defects of Both

Neither MA nor the FEHBP allow the enrollee who chooses a plan with a premium below the premium support level to pocket the difference. In Medicare Advantage the frugal purchaser does get to benefit, but only up to 75 percent of the premium savings (and usually provided in the form of the plan offering "free" Part D benefits). In the FEHBP, the enrollee gets to keep only 25 percent of the savings, with the government reaping the other 75 percent. In real markets, of course, consumers pocket all the savings from their frugal choices.

Reform Needs

Transforming Medicare into a modernized program, based on consumer choice and competition, would require a number of specific policy changes, discussed in more detail elsewhere in this volume. First, Congress would have to update and improve the system of competitive bidding among health plans to establish a fair and efficient government contribution (premium support) on behalf of beneficiaries. Second, Congress would also have to update and improve Medicare's risk adjustment system to eliminate "gaming" of the program at the expense of the taxpayer and to ensure stability in the new consumer-driven market. And finally, Congress should allow maximum flexibility in health benefit offerings, thus stimulating innovation in health care delivery.

Beyond that, Congress should ensure a smooth transition to the new system and maximize the benefits of consumer choice and competition for the entire Medicare population. This would require four major steps:

Grandfather Current Medicare Enrollees

In any transition to a new premium support system, if we assume that the grandfather rule is followed and no benefits are removed from current Medicare enrollees, the default arrangement for them would be to remain in traditional Medicare, in the great majority of cases with a Medigap plan. They should also be given the option to voluntarily enroll in traditional Medicare as improved by the addition of catastrophic coverage, provided they are willing to drop Medigap coverage. This voluntary choice would provide major savings to enrollees without compulsion, and over time their choices would eliminate Medigap and the distortions it creates.

Improve Traditional Medicare to Compete in a Premium Support System

Traditional Medicare should be updated so it can more fairly compete in a premium support system. The most important benefit missing from traditional Medicare is a maximum out-of-pocket limit on hospital and physician costs. Adding it would enable traditional Medicare to compete effectively in a new premium support program, offer potentially massive savings to both enrollees and taxpayers, and eliminate the need to allow new retirees to enroll in Medigap plans. As discussed elsewhere in this book, this and related reforms would be essential to leveling the playing field among competing plans.

End Excess Spending on "Free" Care

A growing body of literature demonstrates that when Medicare enrollees have zero cost sharing for hospital and doctor bills, they consume far more health care than otherwise comparable enrollees. One recent study found that on average Medicare enrollees with Medigap supplement coverage incurred medical claims costs about 33 percent higher for physician care and 24 percent higher for hospital care.[11] Other studies have found similar results.[12]

If Medigap and employer wraparound policies can be replaced with better alternatives voluntarily chosen by retirees, annual cost savings on the order of $2,000 to $3,000 a year per enrollee could be achieved.

About 38 million of the 64 million Medicare enrollees are in traditional Medicare, and about 80 percent of these have either Medigap or employer wraparound policies. Hence, the potential savings from eliminating such wraparounds would be in the range of $80 billion to $120 billion a year after a transition period. This would be more than enough to finance an out-of-pocket limit benefit in traditional Medicare.[13]

Promote Competition When Setting the Government Contribution in a Premium Support System

Coulam, Feldman, and Dowd advocated using the single lowest bid as the basis for a premium support system.[14] Under these or any similar "lowest plan or plans" bid benchmark, ensuing calculations lead to major Medicare savings estimates. Domenici and Rivlin used the cost of the second lowest plan as their benchmark example in 2011, as did a 2017 Congressional Budget Office study.[15]

These are not optimum designs. There are good reasons not to base a premium support system on the lowest individual plan bids, whether the lowest, second lowest, or third lowest. Under a lowest-bid system, plans can make strategic bids (even bids under which they would temporarily lose money) to gain market share, to deprive other plans of market share and force them out of the market, or to otherwise influence bidding and enrollment outcomes. A plan with few enrollees could change the premium support level in ways that disrupt the mainstream market and the performance of the plans that enroll substantial numbers of persons.

The alternative to avoid these problems is to make a fraction of the average bid the basis for the benchmark, the approach used in the FEHBP. Depending on the fraction chosen, any given level of savings or generosity could be achieved. An optimum payment system would be enrollment-weighted and set at a benchmark level that is not significantly different than what multiple lower-cost plans can and do actually achieve while attracting large numbers of enrollees.

Looking Ahead

Medicare premium support, based on the main features outlined here and in other chapters of this book, could work sensibly and effectively. Much would depend on how Washington policymakers design the precise premium and benefit reforms and how they would determine the government contribution to competing health plans. Other authors in this book detail specific measures toward achieving that goal optimally.

Year after year, the Medicare trustees, the Congressional Budget Office, and bipartisan organizations warn that Congress needs to address Medicare's persistent fiscal and programmatic problems. Harnessing the power of consumer choice and improved market competition in Medicare can help resolve those problems. Washington's policymakers must step up to the task.

• •

WALTON J. FRANCIS is an economist and policy analyst who has written and testified on the effectiveness of health insurance programs, including the Federal Employees Health Benefits Program and Medicare, and on potential reforms to those programs, and who pioneered the systematic comparison of health plans for consumers.

NOTES

1. The Medicare Modernization Act of 2003 added a prescription drug benefit to Medicare and mandated catastrophic expense protection in parts of what was renamed Medicare Advantage. Private plan participation in Medicare went through multiple previous incarnations, starting in 1982, but was limited to HMOs until 1997. For a detailed history, see Thomas G. McGuire, Joseph P. Newhouse, and Anna D. Sinaiko, "An Economic History of Medicare Part C," *Milbank Quarterly* 89, no. 2 (2011): 289–332. Other examples of premium support in federal coverage programs include Medicare prescription drug coverage (Part D), which is discussed in detail in chapter 10.

2. Enrollment data from Boards of Trustees of the Federal Hospital Insurance and Federal Supplementary Medical Insurance Trust Funds, *2021 Annual Report of the Boards of Trustees* (Washington, DC: Centers for Medicare and Medicaid Services, August 31, 2021), 157, https://www.cms.gov/files/document/2021 -medicare-trustees-report.pdf.

3. For a detailed comparison of FEHBP and Medicare designs and evolution over time, see McGuire, Newhouse, and Sinaiko, "An Economic History," and Walton Francis, *Putting Medicare Consumers in Charge: Lessons from the FEHBP*

(Washington, DC: American Enterprise Institute (AEI) Press, 2009), https://www
.aei.org/wp-content/uploads/2014/03/-putting-medicare-consumers-in-charge
-book_094528792751.pdf.

4. Henry J. Aaron and Robert D. Reischauer, "The Medicare Reform Debate:
What Is the Next Step," *Health Affairs* 14, no. 40 (1995): 8–30; Stuart M. Butler and
Robert E. Moffit, "The FEHBP as a Model for a New Medicare Program," *Health
Affairs* 14, no. 4 (1995): 47–61.

5. Gail R. Wilensky and Joseph P. Newhouse, "Medicare: What's Right? What's
Wrong? What's Next?," *Health Affairs* 18, no. 1 (1999): 92–106.

6. Mark V. Pauly, *Markets Without Magic: How Competition Might Save Medicare*
(Washington, DC: AEI Press, 2008), https://www.aei.org/wp-content/uploads
/2014/03/-markets-without-magic_102727716432.pdf.

7. Robert F. Coulam, Roger Feldman, and Bryan E. Dowd, *Bring Market Prices to
Medicare: Essential Reform at a Time of Fiscal Crisis* (Washington, DC: AEI Press,
2009), https://www.aei.org/wp-content/uploads/2014/03/-bring-market-prices-to
-medicare_101132912662.pdf.

8. Bipartisan Policy Center, "Testimony by Sen. Pete V. Domenici and Dr. Alice
Rivlin, Co-Chairs, Bipartisan Policy Center Debt Reduction Task Force to the Joint
Select Committee on Deficit Reduction, US Congress," 112th Congress, November 1, 2011, https://www.brookings.edu/wp-content/uploads/2016/06/1101
_deficit_committee_domenici_rivlin-1.pdf.

9. In contrast to Medicare Advantage and marketplace plans under the
Affordable Care Act, most benefits are not specified in detail. In general, medical
services are simply covered if they are medically necessary under normal professional standards for medical care.

10. As discussed in detail in chapter 9 by Edmund F. Haislmaier, Medicare
Advantage also faces opportunities to improve risk adjustment, a different
problem than faced in the FEHBP.

11. Marika Cabral and Neale Mahoney, "Externalities and Taxation of Supplemental Insurance: A Study of Medicare and Medigap," *American Economic Journal:
Applied Economics* 11, no. 2 (2019): 37–73.

12. See also Christopher Hogan, "Exploring the Effects of Secondary Coverage
on Medical Spending for the Elderly" (Washington, DC: Direct Research, August 2014), https://www.medpac.gov/wp-content/uploads/import_data/scrape
_files/docs/default-source/contractor-reports/august2014_secondaryinsurance
_contractor.pdf; US Government Accountability Office (GAO), *Medicare Supplemen-
tal Coverage: Medigap and Other Factors Are Associated with Higher Estimated Health
Care Expenditures*, Report no. GAO-13-811 (Washington DC: GAO, 2013), http://
www.gao.gov/assets/660/657956.pdf; Ezra Golberstein, Kayo Walsh, Yulei He, and
Michael Chernew, "Supplemental Coverage Associated with More Rapid Spending
Growth for Medicare Beneficiaries," *Health Affairs* 32, no. 5 (2013): 873–81,
http://content.healthaffairs.org/content/32/5/873.full.pdf.

13. One recent study addresses the reform problem as it relates to the FEHBP: a
former employer for over 2 million annuitants. There are many options that would

hold enrollees harmless while generating massive savings to Medicare. See Joseph Antos, James C. Capretta, and Walton J. Francis, *Providing High-Quality, Cost-Effective Health Coverage to Retired Federal Employees Age 65 and Older* (Washington, DC: American Enterprise Institute, January 2019), https://www.aei.org/research -products/report/providing-high-quality-cost-effective-health-coverage-to-retired -federal-employees-age-65-and-older.

14. Coulam, Feldman, and Dowd, *Bring Market Prices to Medicare.*

15. Congressional Budget Office, *A Premium Support System for Medicare: Updated Analysis of Illustrative Options* (Washington, DC: Congressional Budget Office, October 2017), https://www.cbo.gov/system/files/115th-congress-2017 -2018/reports/53077-premiumsupport.pdf.

The Potential for Beneficiary and Taxpayer Savings in Moving to a Premium Support Model for Medicare

It is widely appreciated that the United States has a national health spending problem. From 1980 to 2019 total spending rose from $253.2 billion to $3,795.4 billion, an average annual growth of 7.2 percent.[1] Over the same period, gross domestic product (GDP) grew at an average annual rate of 5.3 percent, with the result that national health expenditures rose from 8.9 percent to 17.7 percent of GDP. Thus, in the horse race between costs and the resources to finance those costs, the former have been steadily winning.[2] More recently, the pace has slowed somewhat—it averaged 4.3 percent from 2009 to 2019—but is still outstripping GDP growth.

This problem is mirrored in spending by the Medicare program, which grew from $37.4 billion to $799.4 billion over the 1980–2019 period. Medicare trustees project that spending will grow dramatically from $925.8 billion to $1.849 trillion over the 2020–2031 period.[3] This annual growth rate is fueled by retirement of an increasingly aged population but also by the steady growth of health care costs.[4]

Medicare costs are financed from two sources. The first is taxpayer subsidies in the form of payroll taxes and general revenues. The second is out-of-pocket expenses by beneficiaries to cover their share of premiums, deductibles, co-pays, and the like. Both sources have faced steady upward pressures.

Clearly, the status quo cannot remain unchanged forever, and among the leading candidates for Medicare reform is the premium support model, in part as a way to rein in the cost problems Medicare faces. Premium support would provide a fixed amount of taxpayer resources per beneficiary and could, by definition, be used to reduce the taxpayer contribution to Medicare. The real promise, however, is that the competitive forces embedded in a premium support design would slow the pace of health care cost growth (per beneficiary) in a way that lowers *both* the taxpayer contribution and beneficiary out-of-pocket spending.

This short chapter examines this potential. In what follows, I review the historic performance of Medicare spending growth as well as the sources of these increases. I then turn to the basic design of recent premium support proposals, including a short discussion of key policy decisions underlying the design. I then turn to evidence from previous research and its implications for the potential savings to beneficiaries and taxpayers. The final section is a summary and conclusions.

For policymakers, the primary goal of Medicare reform should be the achievement of better value for this major expenditure of America's health care dollars. Introducing a comprehensive system of premium support in Medicare—broadening both patient choice and a more intensified competition among plans and providers—would enable beneficiaries to act on their values and get the best care and coverage they can that aligns with those values. As a byproduct of this interplay of dynamic market forces, policymakers can feel confident that they will also be able to secure a significant reduction in outlays for both Medicare beneficiaries and federal taxpayers. In any case, a value-driven Medicare program will provide a better social safety net, regardless of its cost.

Trends in Medicare Spending

Under current law, Medicare payroll taxes (1.45 percent each for employers and employees) and the Affordable Care Act payroll surtaxes (3.8 percent of net investment income and 0.9 percent of payroll for high-income individuals) fund Medicare Part A for hospital care. Beneficiaries' premiums cover 25 percent of outpatient care under Medicare Part B, while the remaining is financed by the taxpayer from general revenue. There is a similar 25–75 split of costs in Medicare Advantage (Part C) and the prescription drug program (Part D).

An important feature of this overall design is that Medicare has an unlimited draw on the resources of the American taxpayer, especially through the general revenue provided for Parts B, C, and D. The absence of any effective budget constraint is a fundamental design flaw in Medicare, provides no overall incentives to economize or innovate in the provision of care, and exposes taxpayers and beneficiaries alike to continued upside financial risk.

Consider the numbers from the 2020 report of the Medicare Board of Trustees.[5] In 2019, Medicare spent $796.2 billion on medical services for America's seniors but only collected $400.3 billion in payroll taxes and monthly premiums. This cash shortfall of $396 billion represented 40 percent of the federal deficit in 2019. Indeed, Medicare has had a cash shortfall every year since its creation, except in 1966 and 1974; its cumulative shortfall is $5.5 trillion. As a result, Medicare alone was responsible for 34 percent of all federal debt outstanding at the end of 2019.

A second negative aspect of the current Medicare program is the continual rise in costs per beneficiary. The term "excess cost growth" refers to the fact that health care spending per beneficiary (adjusted for demography) rises faster than GDP per capita. Notice that excess cost growth is a combination of utilization and price increases. Under current law, there are few strong incentives to manage utilization effectively and no competitive forces driving the evolution of prices. As a result, the Congressional Budget Office (CBO) expects excess cost growth in Medicare to continue at an annual rate of 1 percent for the foreseeable future.[6]

Beneficiaries are hardly insulated from these costs. There has been a steady rise the exposure of beneficiaries to out-of-pocket costs (premiums, co-insurance, deductibles, etc.) (see fig. 12.1). Indeed, from 1980 to 2019, the total exposure rose at an average annual rate of 6.2 percent.[7]

What Is Premium Support?

An important aspect of premium support is that it would put Medicare on a budget. Instead of directly paying all of the costs of care in, for example, Parts A and B, under premium support insurers would bid for the right to provide a defined bundle of services to seniors, and the federal government and beneficiary would provide the insurer a fixed contribution. Taxpayer subsidies would be capped and beneficiary premiums would be fixed. Medicare would face a budget constraint, and all the stakeholders (providers, device and drug makers, insurers, and beneficiaries) would shift to a world with strong incentives to control spending.

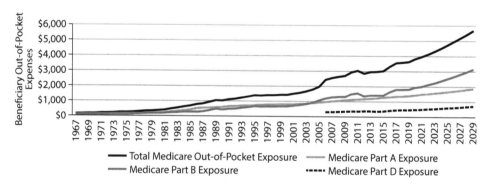

FIGURE 12.1. Medicare Beneficiary Out-of-Pocket Exposure. *Source:* Calculations based on Centers for Medicare and Medicaid Services. Details available upon request from Douglas Holtz-Eakin, President, American Action Forum, 1747 Pennsylvania Avenue, NW, 5th Floor, Washington, DC 20006. Email: dholtzeakin@americanactionforum.org.

The second key aspect is that these amounts are determined by competition among private sector insurers at risk for losses. As a result, those insurers would have strong incentives to offer bids low enough to attract beneficiaries and also keep costs sufficiently low to make a profit. On the flip side, those insurers that are unable to manage their bids and costs successfully will fail in the marketplace.[8]

Unlike the current Medicare system, a premium support approach would embed into the provision of seniors' health care the beneficial dynamism that has characterized the most successful sectors of the US economy.

Key Design Considerations

Not all premium support reforms are created equal; there are some important design considerations that must be contemplated. The first is the scope of the reforms. Will premium support apply solely to the hospital and outpatient benefits in Parts A and B, leaving the existing bidding-based systems in Part C (Medicare Advantage) and Part D (outpatient prescription drugs)?

In the analyses of the Congressional Budget Office, premium support was assumed to affect only Parts A and B, with traditional fee-for-service (FFS) Medicare acting as one plan offering in the bidding process.[9] Medicare Advantage (MA) and Part D, however, use a competitive bidding system (though imperfect) and are an increasingly important part of delivering seniors' health benefits. Today, well over 48 percent of enrollees choose MA. Exposing Part D to an even more competitive bidding system would yield even greater potential savings.

The second important consideration for a premium support design is the geographic area over which competition will take place. One could envision county-level bidding, service area bidding, or other larger geographic area parameters.

Third, one must decide the role of the traditional FFS system. The CBO analyses, for example, envision that the FFS "bid" is automatically set equal to the projected FFS spending for an enrollee of average health in an area. This is a very passive view of the traditional program's role in competition. An alternative would be to empower an agent or trustee to bid on behalf of the traditional FFS, perhaps even lower than the projected spending described above to attract additional beneficiaries.

Fourth, one must pick the mechanism by which the bidding system sets benchmarks, premiums, and subsidies. In its studies, the CBO looked at two possibilities. One was to set the benchmark premium equal to the average bid in the area, while a more aggressive option is to set it equal to the second-lowest bid in the area.

Fifth, there must be a set of rules regarding plan designs and offerings. How many different plans can an insurer offer? What are the limitations on deviations from the actuarial value of the benchmark? These considerations will determine the vigor of competition among insurers and their ability to control offerings with broader and narrower networks of providers.

Finally, there is the issue of the transition to the new system. Will current beneficiaries be grandfathered in their current arrangements, or is the transition to premium support assumed to happen immediately?

Previous Evidence

One source of insight into the impact of a competitive, premium support model is the success of the design of the Medicare Part D program, the existing system of private plans competing to deliver prescription drugs. Since its enactment, the Part D program has continually proven its ability to control beneficiary and budget costs, provide consistently high-quality drug plans, and exemplify market-based competition within an entitlement program.

Established as part of the Medicare Modernization Act of 2003 (MMA), Part D was designed to increase seniors' access to outpatient prescription drugs through the Medicare program. The goal of the policymakers who developed Part D was to provide a stable mechanism for competing insurance issuers to offer prescription drugs at negotiated prices to Medicare beneficiaries.[10] In the past 10 years, the program has more than achieved its goals: costing taxpayers much less than the original budgetary projections, providing a wide variety of low-cost plan options, and maintaining high levels of member satisfaction.[11]

This reliance on genuine private-sector negotiation has worked incredibly well. In fact, total program expenditures have come in far lower than initial CBO projections (see fig. 12.2). Part D's 10-year cost (starting in 2006) was projected in 2004 to be $957.3 billion, after the Medicare Modernization Act was passed but before the program started. By 2011, the combination of five years of actual data and five years of projections totaled $499.4 billion, for a cost *underrun* of $457.9 billion, or about 48 percent. The last CBO forecast for 2012 Part D spending made prior to implementation was in 2005, and the projected 2012 spending in that year was $126.8 billion. After the bids came in for 2006, the 2012 forecast was reduced to $110.2 billion. In all but one of the next six years, the forecast for 2012 was reduced further. The actual amount was $55 billion—about 57 percent lower than the original preimplementation forecast.[12]

The annual Part D bidding process allows issuers to place bids for plans in any or all of the 34 regions in the country. These issuers

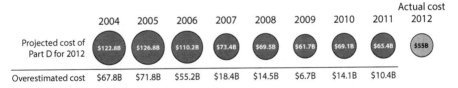

FIGURE 12.2. The Projected Cost of Medicare Part D. *Source:* Calculations are based on Douglas Holtz-Eakin, "Lower Drug Costs Now: Expanding Access to Affordable Health Care," testimony before the Subcommittee on Health, Employment, Labor, and Pensions, Committee on Education and Labor, US House of Representatives, May 5, 2021, https://www.america nationforum.org/testimony/lower-drug-costs-now-expanding-access-to-affordable-health -care.

submit a bid displaying the potential per member per month cost of providing benefits to members in any (or all) of the established regions. All bids contain a rate for the basic benefit, or "standard plan," as well as an enhanced benefit plan that goes above and beyond the minimum plan requirements. Part D members can choose whether they would like to participate in a plan that contracts with nearby pharmacies as part of a preferred provider network, pay a higher premium for plans with enhanced benefits, or save money by selecting a standard plan.

Despite initial worries about plan participation, this process of bidding and selection has led to a large number of available plans; seniors in every region of the country had an average of 30 drug plan choices in 2021.[13]

The open competition for beneficiaries has resulted in a robust market. The ability for plan issuers to negotiate with preferred pharmacy networks, pharmaceutical companies, and pharmacy benefit managers has allowed plans to utilize their market share to obtain lower prices and thus charge lower premiums. For example, a plan may offer drug A at a lower co-payment than an equivalent drug B, and in exchange for doing so they negotiate rebates from the manufacturer of drug A. As a result, patients who have a condition that warrants drug A or B are able to obtain A at a lower out-of-pocket cost, and the Part D plan receives the rebate for every purchase, thus allowing them to price their plan more affordably.

The success of the program is not an accident; Part D is designed to provide seniors with affordable choices. Competitive bidding and plan selection have led to high-quality products, as measured through member satisfaction rates. Despite initial concerns about plan enrollment and member participation in 2020, 92 percent of seniors said that they were satisfied with their Part D coverage,[14] and 87 percent said that their Part D plan delivered good value for the money.[15] The satisfaction reported by seniors displays the use of an efficient, high-quality program that continues to come in under cost projections and maintain popularity among its members.

Another place to look for evidence that the premium support model will be superior to FFS Medicare is to compare it to the performance of the Federal Employees Health Benefits Program (FEHBP).[16] FEHBP has traditionally maintained extremely high levels of enrollee satisfaction, a broad array of plan choices, and moderate growth in costs. FEHBP was part of the inspiration for the successful Part D drug program and continues to demonstrate durable, desirable properties.

Finally, the CBO has issued two reports regarding the impact of a transition to premium support. These reports focus on prototypes of premium support that exclude the dual eligible and participants in Medicare Advantage and the Part D program. In its 2017 update to the analysis, CBO concluded that using the more aggressive second-lowest bid approach to setting the benchmark would reduce both taxpayer costs and beneficiary out-of-pocket costs, the former by 15 percent and the latter by 5 percent. In short, premium support can lower overall spending in the program.

Savings Estimates

I have extrapolated the CBO findings in two ways. First, I applied the savings to all benefits, including MA and Part D (table 12.1). Second, I applied the savings to the 2020 CBO baseline for the Medicare program, augmented with an estimate of the aggregate out-of-pocket costs for the beneficiary population (table 12.2). Overall, total program costs are lowered by 11.5 percent, with savings totaling over $1.8 trillion in taxpayer costs over 10 years and $333 billion in savings to beneficiaries.

These are useful guides to the potential for savings in the program, but they are likely too low. Assigning an agent to bid on behalf of the FFS program in each area would produce more downward pressure on prices; pressure that would affect MA beneficiaries who would no longer be tied to a FFS benchmark.

In addition, insurers could optimize the combination of drug and nondrug therapies to support best medical practice and raise the efficiency of the delivery of all care. Given the importance of Medicare to medical practice patterns overall, this raises the prospect of more systemic competitive pressure on prices and spending throughout the health system.

Finally, and more important than the dollar value of costs savings, the choices made by beneficiaries would identify their desired high-value care. Revealing consumer value by choice in competitive markets has been the foundation of US economic success. Premium sup-

Table 12.1. Baseline Medicare spending (in billions of dollars) by both the traditional program (Parts A, B, and D) and beneficiaries out-of-pocket (OOP)

	2021	2022	2023	2024	2025	2026	2027	2028	2029	2030
Part A	365	405	419	430	475	505	536	591	581	654
Part B	422	474	494	510	574	620	671	759	754	865
Part D	96	111	112	112	131	142	153	178	166	192
Total program spending	883	990	1,025	1,052	1,180	1,267	1,360	1,528	1,501	1,711
OOP spending	470	527	546	560	629	675	725	814	800	912

Sources: Calculations based on Congressional Budget Office (CBO), "Medicare—CBO's Baseline as of March 6, 2020," March 19, 2020, https://www.cbo.gov/system/files/2020-03/51302-2020-03-medicare.pdf; Juliette Cubanski, Wyatt Koma, Anthony Damico, and Tricia Neuman, "How Much Do Medicare Beneficiaries Spend Out of Pocket on Health Care?," Kaiser Family Foundation, November 4, 2019, https://www.kff.org/report-section/how-much-do-medicare-beneficiaries-spend-out-of-pocket-on-health-care-methodology.

Table 12.2. Potential savings (in billions of dollars) from moving to premium support for both the program (benefits) and beneficiaries' out-of-pocket (OOP)

	2021	2022	2023	2024	2025	2026	2027	2028	2029	2030	2021–2030
Benefits savings	132	149	154	158	177	190	204	229	225	257	1,875
OOP savings	24	26	27	28	31	34	36	41	40	46	333
Total savings	156	175	181	186	208	224	240	270	265	303	2,208

Sources: Calculations based on Congressional Budget Office (CBO), "Medicare—CBO's Baseline as of March 6, 2020," March 19, 2020, https://www.cbo.gov/system/files/2020-03/51302-2020-03-medicare.pdf; Juliette Cubanski, Wyatt Koma, Anthony Damico, and Tricia Neuman, "How Much Do Medicare Beneficiaries Spend Out of Pocket on Health Care?," Kaiser Family Foundation, November 4, 2019, https://www.kff.org/report-section/how-much-do-medicare-beneficiaries-spend-out-of-pocket-on-health-care-methodology.

port can introduce this dynamic to Medicare and the health system more generally.

Looking Ahead

On the basis of the evidence to date, there is every reason to expect that a Medicare premium support program can reduce outlays by both beneficiaries and taxpayers, and substantially so. Over the 2022–2031 budget window, for example, Medicare outlays could decline by at least $2.2 trillion, or 11.5 percent. Even more importantly, however, is that the introduction of consumer choice allows beneficiaries to reveal their values on the crucial issue of medical care and coverage. A values-driven Medicare system will be a better social safety net, regardless of its cost.

• •

DOUGLAS HOLTZ-EAKIN is president of the American Action Forum and former director of the Congressional Budget Office.

NOTES

1. All figures taken from the historical data of the Centers for Medicare and Medicaid Services, "2020 National Health Expenditure Data," updated December 15, 2021, https://www.cms.gov/Research-Statistics-Data-and-Systems/Statistics-Trends -and-Reports/NationalHealthExpendData/NationalHealthAccountsHistorical.

2. There is a related, but different, issue of whether current health care spending is delivering high-quality outcomes and is, thus, a good value proposition. I return to this later.

3. Boards of Trustees of the Federal Hospital Insurance and Supplementary Medical Insurance Trust Funds, *2022 Annual Report of the Boards of Trustees* (Washington, DC: Centers for Medicare and Medicaid Services, June 2, 2022), 177, table V.B1, https://www.cms.gov/files/document/2022-medicare-trustees-report.pdf.

4. See Centers for Medicare and Medicaid Services, Office of the Actuary, *The Long-Term Projection Assumptions for Medicare and Aggregate National Health Expenditures* (Washington, DC: Centers for Medicare and Medicaid Services, April 22, 2020), https://www.cms.gov/files/document/long-term-projection -assumptions-medicare-and-aggregate-national-health-expenditures.pdf.

5. All figures taken from Gordon Gray, Tara O'Neill Hayes, and Andrew Strohman, "The Future of America's Entitlements: What You Need to Know about the Medicare and Social Security Trustees Reports," American Action Forum, April 22, 2020, https://www.americanactionforum.org/research/the-future-of

-americas-entitlements-what-you-need-to-know-about-the-medicare-and-social
-security-trustees-reports-3, and author's calculations.

6. CBO, *The 2021 Long-Term Budget Outlook* (Washington, DC: Congressional Budget Office, March 2021), 22, https://www.cbo.gov/system/files/2021-03/56977 -LTBO-2021.pdf.

7. Author's calculations based on data cited in note 1.

8. Importantly, this competition occurs at the plan level. Thus, the savings discussed herein are not the result of reforming consumer incentives (e.g., reform of Medigap policies). CBO assumes no change in Medigap rules in its analyses.

9. CBO, *A Premium Support System for Medicare: Analysis of Illustrative Options* (Washington, DC: Congressional Budget Office, September 2013), https://www.cbo .gov/publication/44581; CBO, *A Premium Support System for Medicare: Updated Analysis of Illustrative Options* (Washington, DC: Congressional Budget Office, October 2017), https://www.cbo.gov/publication/53077.

10. *Medicare Prescription Drug, Improvement, and Modernization Act of 2003*, H.R. 1, 108th Congress, enacted December 8, 2003, Section 101, https://www.congress .gov/bill/108th-congress/house-bill/1.

11. Robert A. Book and Douglas Holtz-Eakin, "Competition in the Medicare Part D Program," American Action Forum, September 11, 2013, https://www .americanactionforum.org/research/competition-and-the-medicare-part-d-program.

12. Hanns Kuttner, "Introductory Essay," in *The Medicare Drug Benefit Five Years Later: Is It Working?*, edited by Hanns Kuttner and Tevi Troy (Washington, DC: Hudson Institute, December 2011), 7, https://www.hudson.org/content /researchattachments/attachment/990/themedicaredrugbenefit--dec2011.pdf.

13. Juliette Cubanski and Anthony Damico, "Medicare Part D: A First Look at Medicare Prescription Drug Plans in 2021," Kaiser Family Foundation, October 29, 2020, https://www.kff.org/medicare/issue-brief/medicare-part-d-a-first-look-at -medicare-prescription-drug-plans-in-2021.

14. Morning Consult, "Results: Medicare Part D Recipients' Perceptions of Care," July 2021, 1, http://medicaretoday.org/wp-content/uploads/2021/07 /2106179_HLC_Medicare-Part-D_Satisfaction_7.27.21_final.pdf.

15. Medicare Today, "2020 Senior Satisfaction Survey," accessed November 8, 2021, https://medicaretoday.org/resources/senior-satisfaction-survey; Morning Consult, "More than 90 Percent of Seniors Are Satisfied with Medicare Part D," accessed November 8, 2021, http://medicaretoday.org/wp-content/uploads/2020 /08/MT_2020-Senior-Satisfaction-Survey-Fact-Sheet.pdf.

16. For a good summary of this, see *Competition in a Modernized Medicare: Separating Fact from Fiction*, hearing before the Senate Special Committee on Aging, 108th Congress (2003), testimony of Walton Francis, accessed September 23, 2021, https://www.aging.senate.gov/imo/media/doc/hr99wf.pdf. See also Stuart Butler and Robert E. Moffit, "The FEHBP as a Model for a Medicare New Program," *Health Affairs* 14, no. 4 (1995): 47–61, https://www.healthaffairs.org /doi/abs/10.1377/hlthaff.14.4.47.

39–42, 47–49, 144, 203–4; financing of, 7–8, 201–2, 203–4; governance of, 134; impact of changes to, 31–34; impact of demographic shifts on, 5; impact of the COVID pandemic on, 42, 49; insurance design of, 85–86;; medical outcomes under, 60–61; Medicare Advantage as model for reform of, 114–18; need for reform of, 1–2, 8–18, 34–35, 36–37, 43, 47; original version of, 189; payment rates as compared with private insurance rates, 41–42; popularity of, 27; prescription drug coverage under, 2, 8, 16–17, 19, 62–73, 90, 109; problems inherent in, 19–20; public choice approach to, 27–31, 35–37; role of private plans in, 89–90; special needs plans (SNPs) under, 90, 94–95, 97, 98, 114; structural reforms to, 109; structure of, 3–4; supplemental coverage under, 5–6, 10, 40, 81, 194; sustainability of, 85; transition to modernized Medicare, 133–34; unfunded obligations of, 6. *See also* defined contribution plans; Medicare Advantage; Medicare, recommendations for reform of